A Just Minimum of Health Care

A JUST MINIMUM OF HEALTH CARE

Kenneth F. T. Cust

University Press of America, Inc.
Lanham • New York • Oxford

Copyright © 1997 by
University Press of America,® Inc.
4720 Boston Way
Lanham, Maryland 20706

12 Hid's Copse Rd.
Cummor Hill, Oxford OX2 9JJ

Library of Congress Cataloging-in-Publication Data

Cust, Kenneth F. T.
A just minimum of health care / Kenneth F. T. Cust.
p.   cm.
Includes bibliographical references and index.
1. Right to health care--United States. 2. Right to health care--
Canada. 3. Social contract. 4. Social Justice. I. Title.
RA394.C885 1997   362.1'0973--dc21 97-12077 CIP

ISBN 0-7618-0753-5 (cloth: alk. ppr.)
ISBN 0-7618-0754-3 (pbk: alk. ppr.)

⊖™ The paper used in this publication meets the minimum
requirements of American National Standard for information
Sciences—Permanence of Paper for Printed Library Materials,
ANSI Z39.48—1984

Contents

Preface

Increasing numbers of Americans are uninsured, the cost of health care is escalating, and is projected to continue doing so. In response to these and other concerns, Americans have looked to their neighbor to the north, Canada, for possible help in treating the ills of America's health care system. In addition to offering a comparative analysis of the Canadian and American health care systems, we have sought to identify the facts that motivte concerns on both sides of the border. It is within this larger context, we argued, that the question of justice in health care must be answered.

We consider two alternative answers that have been advanced in response to the question of justice in health care, Norman Daniels' fair equality of opportunity argument and Allen Buchanan's enforced beneficence arguments for a right to a decent minimum of health care. After subjecting these arguments to critical scrutiny, we found that they could not bear the moral weight that the authors thought they could.

We then considered an alternative account that might be used to address the question of justice in health care, David Gauthier's theory of justice. We concluded, among other things, that under his theory people would have a right to a just minimum of health care. In addition, we argued that a just minimum of health care would resolve the theory-dependent version of the bottomless pit problem.

Acknowledgement

The author wishes to acknowledge all those people who lent their support, guidance, and efforts toward the completion of this project. Special appreciation is extended to R. G. Frey, Loren Lomasky, Edward F. McClennen, Fred D. Miller, Jr., Denise Trauth, and extra special appreciation is extended to Christopher Morris. I should also like to thank David Gauthier who read an early draft of Chapter VI. In addition, I should also like to thank the Directors of the Social Philosophy & Policy Center, Fred D. Miller, Jr., Ellen Frankel Paul, and Jeffrey Paul, for their support over the past few years, the H. B. Earhart Foundation for two years of financial support, and the Center of Medical Ethics at the University of Pittsburgh for giving me the opportunity to spend a semester doing research and gaining clinical experience in medical ethics. There were several scholars who passed through the Social Philosophy and Policy Center who gave me the opportunity to discuss my ideas with them: Norman Barry, Anthony Flew, John Gray, Roderick T. Long, and David Schmidtz. I would also like to thank my wife Fran, my family, and friends for their encouragement and support. Finally, I would like to thank my brother Nelson for his assistance in preparing the final draft of the manuscript.

Parts of chapters 1 through 6 draw on material that originally appeared in *Reason Papers* 18 (Fall, 1993).

Chapter 1

The Question of Justice in Health Care

While the question of justice could be raised about many different aspects of health care, we will restrict our concern to the practice of medicine and the different social institutions and structures Canada and the United States have thus far endorsed for the delivery and provision of health care to their respective citizens. More specifically we will be concerned with the issues of moral rights to health care, the extent and limitations of these rights, and the implications such moral rights would have for the social institutions constructed to deliver health care in these two countries. Conceptually one could approach the question of justice in health care from one of several different philosophical perspectives, egalitarianism, utilitarianism, libertarianism, or contractarianism. The approach taken here is contractarian, and more specifically, the contractarianism recently argued for by David Gauthier in his *Morals by Agreement.* Our main thesis is that people do have a moral right to health care; that is, we shall argue that people are entitled to what we shall call a just minimum of health care.

Given the nature of our proposed inquiry, three questions come immediately to mind. Why conduct the proposed inquiry using Gauthier's theory of justice? Why Canada and the United States, especially given the difference between the health care systems in these countries, not to mention numerous and substantial cultural, geographic, and demographic differences? And why focus principally on the issue of rights to health care when there are other, perhaps even more pressing, bioethical issues? These are important questions for they force us to consider not only the nature of our proposed inquiry, but also what motivates it.

Our reasons for adopting Gauthier's theory of justice in this inquiry are threefold. First, the theory of justice advanced by Gauthier is important for it is based on four important notions central to contemporary (as well as classical) liberal moral, and political theory: namely the notions of liberty, equality, consent, and mutual advantage. Second, to the extent that Gauthier's theory of justice is defensible, then, as we will argue in Chapters VI and VII, it has profound implications for the doctor-patient relationship, how we structure the delivery of health care, the rights people have as consumers of health care, and the rights people have as providers of health care. Finally, the theory of justice articulated by Gauthier makes an important contribution to our understanding of morality, the nature and scope of our obligations to our fellow man, and it provides us with yet another moral framework from which we can view the world in general and our health care institutions in particular.

A comparative analysis of Canadian and American health care delivery systems will be instructive, and not only for the reason that many Americans are looking north to their neighbor for guidance in diagnosing and treating the ills of the American system of health care delivery. Canadians too are looking, as well as coming, south to the United States when they reach (and are unable to breach) the boundaries imposed by Canada's system of health care delivery (Barnes 1990, p. A16). Furthermore, as some health care consumers in both countries are just beginning to realize, and which will be documented in what follows, what might be called the meta-structure of health care -- that is, the profession of medicine itself -- is becoming increasingly suspect, and principally for the reason that the profession of medicine has failed to "return itself to a fiduciary agency from which it has wandered over the past two decades" (Wolinsky 1988, p. 44). Thus a comparative analysis will give health care consumers in both countries not only an opportunity to learn both the strengths and weaknesses of each other's system of health care delivery, but also the opportunity to grasp the nature and source of the deficiency of the meta-structure of health care.

The question of whether or not there is a moral right to health care is also important, and for a number of reasons. Health care is important, for not only can it mean the difference between life and death, it can also affect the quality of one's life. In addition, if we can answer the question of whether or not people have a moral right to health care, we may also be in a position to resolve some other medical/ethical problems. For example, there is the problem of having limited health care resources and a virtually unlimited need for health care. This problem, commonly called the "bottomless pit" problem (Fried 1978, chap. 5; Daniels 1985, p. 53), can be resolved if we know what people are morally entitled to with respect to health care. Suppose people are, as we shall argue, entitled to a just minimum of health care. If people are entitled to a just minimum of health care, then we shall be in a position to determine whether or not they are entitled to a specific health care procedure. On our account, people would be entitled to all those health care procedures the sum of which do not exceed the just minimum. One should not interpret this latter claim to mean that people could only consume the just minimum of health care and no more. On our account, as we shall argue, all people have a moral right to a just minimum of health care and they would be morally entitled to consume the just minimum; in addition, if they could pay for it, they would be legally entitled to consume more health care.

In discussing the issue of rights to health care, we first need to be clear on what rights are. While we could digress and consider some of the more substantive philosophical disagreements about rights, we will not. For, as Sumner rightly notes, everyone agrees that whatever rights may be, they give normative advantages (Sumner 1987, p. 32). However, we do need at least a working account of the concept of a right. Rights, be they moral or legal rights, involve obligations. If one person has a right, then this implies an obligation on the part of at least one other person. On this view, to say that S has a right to X is to imply that someone has an obligation to S to either provide S with X or to refrain from restricting S's liberty to pursue X. If one is obligated to provide S with X, we say S has a positive right to X. On the other hand, if S is under no obligation not to do X, then we say S has a negative right to X or a right not to be interfered with in the pursuit of X, or in short, a liberty.

The distinction between a positive right and a negative right is important to our argument. If we fail to make clear this distinction, our position may be misinterpreted; that is, if we apply this account of what it is to have a right to the issue of rights to health care and we fail to keep this distinction in mind, then we may be understood to be saying one of two things. On the one hand, we could be interpreted to mean that people have a positive right to health care. On the other hand, we could be interpreted to mean that people have the negative right not to have their liberty restricted in caring for their own health. To minimize the possibility of misinterpretation in what follows, we shall refer to these different senses of rights as, respectively, a positive right and a negative right. If we now apply this distinction to our central thesis -- that is that people have a moral right to a just minimum of health care -- we can be understood to mean that people have a positive right to a just minimum of health care.

The thesis that people do have a positive right to a just minimum of health care must, of course, be defended. However, before defending this thesis, we must first consider the larger context of our health care institutions in which such claims of justice are advanced. For it is within the larger context of our health care institutions that claims of justice in health care need to be adjudicated. In addition, the question of justice in health care must take into account both the health care institutions and the practices of health care providers to determine, at least in part, what constitutes justice in health care.

The systems of health care delivery in Canada and the United States differ in many respects, as we shall see in the following chapter, but they are also similar in many respects. In both countries physicians are the main providers of medical care; that is, in both countries physicians have been granted a monopoly on the practice of medical care. (We shall consider Kenneth Arrow's justification for granting physicians this monopoly in Chapter VI.) Physicians, as an organized body of health care practitioners and through their respective professional organizations, define what constitutes medical care, what practices are medical practices, and what treatments or procedures are medical treatments and/or procedures. In both countries physicians have enormous social prestige, political power, wealth, and privileges. And while the health care institutions in both Canada and the United States may be the envy of lessor developed countries, they are not without problems. Health care consumers have become increasingly alarmed by the rising costs of health care in Canada and especially in the United States. In the United States there is also concern about the ever increasing number of uninsured and underinsured. There is concern about the amount of unnecessary and inappropriate care, the incidence of iatrogenic (or an unintentional injury caused by a physician) injuries, the amount of nosocomial infections (infections contracted while in hospital), and the subsequent economic costs of these practices. There is also concern about the phenomenon of physician-induced demand for medical care, the amount and cost of medical fraud, the problem of self-referral and physician ownership of medical diagnostic and therapeutic centers and equipment. These concerns, which will be discussed in more detail below, have led to dissatisfaction for many Canadians and Americans. Moreover, some academics view these events as precipitating the decline of medicine as a profession.

In addition to these reasons, Haug argues that the profession of medicine is in decline for different reasons: the popularization of medical knowledge, the increasing specialization of medicine, the erosion of physician autonomy, "the acid test of professional status" (Wolinski 1988, p. 44), the erosion of physician authority over patients due to the gradual displacement of the beneficence model of the physician-patient relationship by the autonomy model (Beauchamp and McCullough, 1984, pp. 22-51). Haug also cites the role of computers in deprofessionalizing medicine. Personal computers have penetrated both the home and schools, and children are now introduced to computers at a very early age and continue to use them. People who do not know how to use computers are referred to as computer illiterate. Thus, with respect to the issue of medical knowledge in general and medical care in particular, which Pauly argues is "almost as much a market for information as it is a market for specific services" (Pauly 1988, p. 228), Haug concludes that "in a period when second graders are operating personal computers in school, the time may come when the issue will not be who has the knowledge in her brain, but who knows the technique for extracting it" (Haug 1988, p. 51).[1]

Computer programs can already outperform doctors diagnostically in certain areas. In a recent study a computer had a 97% success rate at diagnosing heart attacks compared to the doctors in the study, who had a success rate of only 78% (Waldholz 1991,

p. A7). Some computer programs, for example, APACHE (Acute Physiology Assessment and Chronic Health Evaluation), are also being used at the bedside to predict patient outcomes (Donaldson 1992, p. 48cc). There currently exist several computer programs that can diagnose large numbers of diseases; for example, ILIAD, a computer program, can diagnose over 1300 medical problems. In addition, computers can and are being used to teach anatomy, physiology, and pathophysiology; for example, ANATOMIST, a CD-ROM multimedia database of human anatomy, has over 500 anatomical illustrations and 2500 medical terms with definitions. A.D.A.M. (Animated Dissection of Anatomy for Medicine) is a fully interactive software program so that people can simulate surgery and other medical procedures (Barron 1992, pp. 20-27; Harrison 1992, pp. 16-19). Finally, should one wish to increase one's knowledge about the potential side effects of various prescription and nonprescription drugs, one can simply use a computer to tie into the Food and Drug Administration's database to get the latest information on virtually any drug in use in the United States (Nelson 1992, p. 17). While such software may be available the AMA has already given advance warning that if software companies begin to market such software directly to health care consumers "that action may violate the medical licensing laws" (Andrews 1986, p. 6).

One might want to object that computers cannot replace physicians for at least two different reasons. First, one might argue that current computer programs are insufficiently sophisticated to replace physicians. Second, one might argue that even if computer programs do attain the requisite degree of sophistication, they would still be unable to bestow on the patient the caring that is a crucial part of the physician's contribution to medical care. One can grant both these objections and still make the case that, in the first place, even if computer programs are not now sufficiently sophisticated to replace physicians, they soon will be. In addition, computers may not replace physicians but they might be used as a diagnostic tool by either physicians or nonphysicians to further one's knowledge about medical care. Finally, even if we assume that computers could never bestow the ethos of caring to patients, some patients may be content without it. That is, some patients may be indifferent to what diagnoses them, a physician or a computer, and sometimes they may prefer the latter to the former. In either case, if computers were sufficiently sophisticated, then, at the very least, patients would have an alternative that they now do not have.

Light and Levine argue, in support of Haug's position on the deprofessionalization of medicine, that the proletarianization or deprofessionalization of medicine[2] is "the trend of the future" (Light *et al*, 1998. p. 14). Stoeckle has concluded that if the profession of medicine is in decline, as Coburn has argued is most certainly the case in Canada (Coburn 1988, p. 111), then while it may no longer be the profession it once was, it at least stands a chance as emerging as a "good job" (Stoeckle 1988, p. 89). Friedson's position on professions is that they emerge and achieve the dominance they ultimately rise to primarily on the basis of the public's perception that they will subscribe to and maintain the fiduciary responsibility of their professional ethic (Friedson 1986, chap. 2). On the eve of the 21st century the public's perception that the profession of medicine has lived up to its professional ethic, "medicine's original avowed promise" (Wolinsky 1988, p. 45), has become increasingly suspect, and for several reasons.

Anecdotal evidence from the media has played some role in the public's diminishing respect for the profession of medicine (Altman 1992, Section 1, p. 1; Kotulak 1985, Section 2, p. 5; Beck 1985a, Section 1, p. 14; Beck 1985b, Section 1, p. 12; Winslow 1992, p. B1; Anderson and Van Atta, 1991, Section D, p. 8; Stout 1992a, p. B5; Crenshaw 1991, Section H, p. 3). For example, the public has recently learned that 7 patients died and 185 others suffered serious complications from inadequately trained physicians performing laparoscopic cholecystectomies (gallbladder removal using a laparoscope, an endoscope equipped for viewing the abdominal cavity through a small incision and performing local surgery) (Altman 1992, p. A1). While this particular incident of iatrogenic injuries received wide media coverage, there are an increasing number of reputable scientific studies available to academics and policy makers indicating that physicians have neither met nor maintained their professional responsibilities when it comes to the health and well-being of their patients. And it is this latter evidence that is most disturbing, for it is ultimately responsible for the gradual erosion of confidence, or as the AMA sees it, the "crisis in confidence" (Todd 1992, p. 98) that the American and Canadian public have in its health care providers and the additional costs these providers force on health care consumers.

For example, a recent study has demonstrated that handwashing by hospital personnel, including medical, nursing, and technical personnel, is "one of the simplest and most important interventions" (Doebbeling *et al*, 1992, p. 92) for reducing the number and cost of nosocomial infections. Nosocomial infections are responsible for a direct annual cost of $5 billion to $10 billion to the U.S. health care system, not including their contribution to morbidity and mortality rates (Doebbeling *et al*, p. 92). Yet, despite the ease by which the number of such infections could be reduced by simply washing one's hand between patient contacts, hospital personnel have consistently failed to do so. Their failure to act in the face of such evidence not only increases the economic cost of health care, it also unnecessarily places patients at risk for increased morbidity and mortality.

A noted Harvard study found that adverse events[3] ensued in 3.7% of hospitalizations. Of these adverse events, 27.6% were due to negligence. Of the adverse events that were due to negligence, 70.5% resulted in a disability lasting less than six months, while 2.6% caused permanently disabling injuries, and 13.6% resulted in death (Brennan *et al*, February 7, 1991, p. 370). The conclusion drawn from this study was "there is a substantial amount of injury to patients from medical management, and many injuries are the result of substandard care" (Brennan *et al*, February 7, 1991, p. 370). Another study estimated that in 1984, in the state of New York alone, the total cost of iatrogenic injuries was $878 million in 1989 dollars (Johnson *et al*, 1992, p. 2492).

Other recent studies have demonstrated an increasing incidence of fraud by physicians. Estimates range from 10% to 25% of the $66 billion the state and federal government spends on Medicaid (Jesilow *et al*, 1991, p. 3318), and it is reported that the U.S. General Accounting Office estimates that "only a fraction of the health insurance fraud and abuse that occurs is identified" (Insurance Fraud Usually Not Spotted, Report Says, 1992, p. 41). Similar estimates indicate that insurance fraud costs the U.S. health care consumer some $55 billion a year (Garcia 1989, p. 49) and that if continued unchecked could amount to $100 billion by 1995 (Fraud Seen Accounting for 10% of Healthcare Spending, 1992, p. 12).[4] A recent General Accounting Office study, in reviewing 500 private psychiatric hospital cases, found that in 64% of the cases reviewed the costs, "hundreds of millions of dollars," could not be justified (Texas Near End of Psychiatric Hospital Chain Probe, 1992, p. 56).

In addition to the problems of nosocomial infections, iatrogenic injuries, and fraud is the problem of physician self-referral; that is, physicians who refer their patients for tests at labs and centers in which they have a direct or indirect financial interest. A recent Florida study[5] has shown that 149 of the 160 diagnostic imaging centers in the state of Florida, or 93.2%, have physician owners. Physicians also own 80% of the radiation therapy centers, 75% of the ambulatory surgical facilities, just over 60% of the clinical laboratories and nearly 40% of the physical therapy rehabilitation centers (Mitchell and Scott, 1992, pp. 82-83). Florida is not unique in having health care facilities owned by physicians.[6] In California, of the 187 freestanding centers that offer magnetic resonance imaging (MRI) services, 85% have physician owners. In the state of New Jersey 75% of the freestanding MRI centers are owned by physicians (Mitchell and Scott, 1992, p. 84). Ownership of such services by physicians is not (or at least need not be) a problem. The problem arises when these owner-physicians initiate self-referrals.

In summarizing the conclusions reached in the 1991 Florida Health Care Cost Containment Board study, Crane noted that the patients of those physicians who had invested in clinical laboratories were the recipients of 45% more clinical laboratory services than all Medicaid patients (Crane 1992, p. 86). These doctor-owned laboratories also conducted "almost twice as many diagnostic tests and received over twice as much in gross revenues per patient as similar non-joint venture facilities" (Crane 1992, p. 86). With respect to MRIs in Florida, residents of Jacksonville, Miami, and Orlando received 14%, 65%, and 35% more services, respectively, than statistically comparable citizens of Baltimore (Crane 1992, p. 86). And again, the residents of these three cities received, respectively, 5.4%, 27.9%, and 14.3% more CT (computer topography) scans than their statistically comparable counterparts in Baltimore (Crane 1992, p. 86). And finally "physician ownership resulted in 27% more home health visits per patient and from 35% to 43% more physical therapy visits per patient" (Crane 1992, p. 86). Dr. Sidney Wolfe, head of the Public Citizen Health Research Group in Washington, estimated that "in Florida alone, this leads to

$500 million in unnecessary tests each year" (Burton 1992, p. B12)[7], not to mention the costs patients suffered in time, opportunity, and iatrogenic injuries due to these unnecessary tests. In addition to the aforementioned costs, there is the moral problem of unnecessary diagnostic and treatment procedures being performed on patients without their informed consent.[8]

Further studies have provided even more evidence that when physicians own the facilities to which they refer their patients, both frequency of testing and cost of testing is substantially higher than referrals by non-owner physicians. One such study found that "the self-referring physicians obtained imaging examinations 4.0 to 4.5 times more than the radiologist-referring [or non-owner] physician" (Hillman *et al*, 1990, p. 1604). With respect to charges for the imaging services rendered, this same study found that the "mean imaging charges per episode of care [...] were 4.4 to 7.5 times higher for the self-referring physician" (Hillman *et al*, 1990, p. 1604). In yet another study by the Department of Health and Human Services, and which was acknowledged by the AMA's Council on Ethical and Judicial Affairs when it recently reconsidered the issue of physician self-referral, researchers found that patients were referred for clinical laboratory testing at a 45% higher rate by self-referring physicians than by non-self-referring physicians (AMA Council on Ethical and Judicial Affairs 1992, p. 2367).[9] In Canada one study found that not only did costs for diagnostic services rise faster that the consumer price index, but that one "laboratory had cost increases (in real terms) of 162 percent between 1971 and 1981" (Crichton *et al*, 1990, p. 92).[10] The results of these American studies have been replicated in further studies. Hillman *et al* recently replicated their original study and concluded that

> the essential result remains unchanged; physicians who own imaging technology employ diagnostic imaging in the evaluation of their patients significantly more often and, as a result, generate 1.6 to 6.2 times higher average imaging charges per episode of care than do physicians who refer imaging examinations to radiologists (Hillman *et al*, 1992, p. 2054).

Another study examined physician ownership of physical therapy services. The main conclusion drawn in this study was that "visits per patient were 39% to 45% higher in joint venture facilities. Both gross and net revenue per patient were 30% to 40% higher in facilities owned by referring physicians"

(Mitchell and Scott, 1992, p. 2055). In addition, this latter study also found that in physical therapy clinics that were owned by physicians, licensed physical therapists spent "on average about 28 minutes of their time per patient visit" (Mitchell and Scott, 1992, p. 2058). In contrasting these results with licensed physical therapists operating in facilities that were not owned by physicians, it was found that therapists in these facilities averaged "72% more time per visit (an average of 48 minutes per visit) treating patients" (Mitchell and Scott, 1992, p. 2058). With respect to utilization, this latter study found that physician-owned physical therapy clinics averaged "about 50% more visits per year than their non-joint venture counterparts" (Mitchell and Scott, 1992, p. 2057). Two additional studies provide further support for the thesis that physician self-referrals significantly increase the cost of health care. The first study found that costs and volume of usage in free standing radiotherapy clinics were 40% to 60% higher in self-referral clinics (Mitchell and Sunshine, 1992, pp. 1497-1501). The second study found that self-referring physicians referred patients for physical therapy 2.3 times more often than non-self-referring physicians and that self-referring physicians ordered unnecessary (as determined by an independent review firm) MRI scans 36% more often than non-self-referring physicians. Another finding of this latter study was that psychiatric evaluations ordered by self-referring physicians was 26% more expensive than that offered by non-self-referring physicians (Swedlow *et al*, 1992, pp. 1502-1506).

Other studies, on the sources of growth in physician expenditures for Medicare, also give cause for concern. In one such study the authors noted that "while office and hospital visits have not been growing particularly fast, more detailed analysis suggests the occurrence of upcoding or procedure-coding creep" (Berenson and Holahan, 1992, p. 688).[11] The study found that during the period studied, 1985 through 1988, while the number of services and allowed charges for the code with the lowest reimbursement rate (the brief office visit) declined 8.3% and 4.9% respectively, the number of services and the allowed charges for the code with the highest reimbursement rate, the extended office visit, increased by 13.2% and 19.8% respectively (Berenson and Holahan, 1992, p. 688). The authors also observed that there was a similar pattern of movement toward billing for higher priced visits in other sites of service, including the emergency department, nursing home, and the home. They concluded that the "consistency of altered coding patterns in all settings suggests, but does not prove, that the pattern of physicians' claims represents procedure-coding creep and not a different case mix of patients" (Berenson and Holahan, 1992, p. 689). A second study, which focused on Medicare's Part B, found that

> In fiscal year 1987, Medicare Part B, the bulk of which is physicians' services, cost $30.8 billion, an increase of 17.5% over the previous years, making it one of the fastest growing federal social programs (McMenamin 1988, p. 94).

The findings of this latter study raises the ethical and financial issue of physician-induced demand for medical services.[12]

There are two components to the issue of physician-induced demand for medical services, the empirical and the theoretical. While we will not concern ourselves with the theoretical component,[13] on the empirical front there is a multitude of evidence from both Canada and the United States that physicians (as well as dentists)[14] indeed induce demand for their services, thus not only greatly increasing the cost of physician-supplied services but also placing uniformed and unconsenting patients at risk for iatrogenic injuries due to the complications of many of these services. Reinhardt decomposes the problem of physician-induced demand into three components. (1) Can physicians manipulate their patient's demand for physician services? (2) If so, do physicians ever do this for the sake of pecuniary gain? And (3), If so, will physicians at any time have fully exploited the potential to maximize their hourly income in this way, or is there unexploited slack whose extent varies with the economic pressure on the physician (Reinhardt 1985, p. 189)? Economists, as theoreticians, typically focus on the third question. We do not maintain that physicians are maximizers with respect to income. While physicians may not be maximizers with respect to income, they may operate according to what has been called the "target-income hypothesis" (Farley 1986, p. 317; Evans 1974). That is, physicians may strive to maintain an income level which they believe they deserve, despite cost-containment policies of health care consumers, business, and/or government.

The seminal study on physicians inducing demand was Fuchs' study of surgeons. In that study he concluded that

> where surgeons are more numerous, the demand for operations

increases. Other things equal, a 10 percent higher surgeon population ratio results in about a 3 percent increase in the number of operations and an increase in price. Thus, the average surgeon's workload decreases by 7 percent, but income per surgeon declines by much less (Fuchs 1978, p. 54).

In addition to Fuchs' study, several other studies reached similar conclusions. A 1970 study on operations and surgeons in the United States and England and Wales found that not only were there twice as many surgeons in the United States, but also that they did twice as many operations (Bunker 1970, p. 135). The amount of surgery in U.S. hospitals continues to increase. Between 1972 and 1981 the number of hospital cases involving surgery increased by 49%. Particular surgical procedures showed dramatic increases: hip arthroplasties (or total hip replacement) were up by 244%; coronary artery surgery was up by 419%; surgery for obesity was up by 132%; and cataract surgery was up 207% (Sloan *et al*, 1986, pp. 31-32). With respect to the diffusion of surgical technology, it was found that the diffusion of such technology was "more likely to occur in markets which the more generous payers predominate" (Sloan *et al*, 1986, p. 31). This result is consistent, as one economist observed, "with the general economic notion that entrepreneurs will innovate if they expect the change to be profitable" (Lewit 1986, p. 99). A recent study on surgeons concluded that "the Medicare program is paying physicians considerably more for many operations than their resource costs would justify" (Mitchell *et al*, 1987, p. 127). An alternate view is that there are fewer surgeons doing fewer operations and that that will lead to a "crisis of unprecedented proportions" -- because they will be lacking in surgical technique -- and that "if 1987 seems bad, then 1997 might prove a disaster" (Rutkow 1987, p. 88).

In a study of physician expenditures in both Canada and the United States, Fuchs and colleagues concluded, among other things, that the higher use rates of medical services by Canadians could be "explained by demand induced by Canadian physicians" (Fuchs *et al*, 1990, p. 888). In a study that analyzed the results of several other studies on the effects of either increasing, freezing, and decreasing reimbursements to physicians, the authors concluded that "these studies show that freezing or reducing payment levels is not effective in controlling program expenditures, because physicians respond by increasing the quantity and complexity of services provided" (Gabel and Rice, 1985, p. 595; Rice

1987, pp. 375-376). Another study concluded by stating that "observed utilization rates are almost exclusively determined by physician supplies (surgeons per thousand); fees and most socio-economical factors have no discernible effect" (Cromwell and Mitchell, 1986, p. 309). Another study, using Canadian data, concludes that "physicians can, and do, generate demand in response to real fee reductions" (Rice and Labelle, 1989, p. 595). In yet another study covering 1983 through 1986, a period in which Medicare fees were frozen, the authors found that

> While the trend in quantity was initially flat at the start of the freeze (Q3-Q4 in 1984), services subsequently grew so that by the end of 1986 (the end of the freeze) quantity per beneficiary was $24 greater (in 1983 dollars) than at the beginning of the freeze, a 21 percent increase.

> Physicians per capita, on the other hand, grew only 1.6 percent over the period of the freeze in our four states, so that quantities per physician rose nearly 20 percent (21% - 1.6% = 19.4%) over the freeze interval (Wedig *et al*, 1989, p. 613).

They concluded their study with the rather startling and strong recommendation that "physicians must be put directly at risk for the cost of their practice style;" in other words, "physicians may need to be placed increasingly at financial risk for at least some of the services they provide" (Wedig *et al*, 1989, p. 617). And again, "analyses of the U.S. experience with fee freezes in the early 1970s clearly demonstrates that increased billing occurred as a response" (Evans *et al*, 1989, p. 575).

Studies in Canada have also demonstrated the effect of physicians inducing demand, notwithstanding provincial attempts to control fees.[15] In one study involving both Quebec and British Columbia, the results were staggering, and left the author concluding that "over the whole period from 1971 to the mid-1980s, the Canadian experience provides support for the hypothesis that utilization per physician increases to offset controls on fees" (Barer *et al*, 1988, p. 16). The most important findings of this study are summarized below.

> To summarize the aggregate Quebec experience with universal medical insurance: over fourteen years fees rose 73 percent (all since 1975), but in real terms (relative to the Consumer Price Index) they actually fell 43 percent! Utilization per capita, however, rose by a remarkable 88 percent, so that real cost per capita actually rose slightly (0.5 percent per year). This rapid increase in

utilization, combined with the increase in fees after 1976, raised fee payments per capita by 225 percent over the fourteen years (Barer *et al*, 1988, p. 31).

In summary, British Columbia's physicians fared relatively well over the period from 1974/1975 to 1983/1984, gaining fee increases exceeding the general inflation rate of 1 percent per year. At the same time the potential supply of patients per physician was falling about 1.5 percent per year. Yet, service provision per physician rose 2 percent per year. This is, in fact, slightly higher than the rate over the same period for Quebec, but considerably lower than the Quebec experience from 1971 to 1976 (Barer *et al*, 1988, p. 38).

One should note that in Quebec, beginning in 1976, fee controls were in place. They lapsed in 1980 but were resumed in 1981. During that one year lapse billings grew 5.18%, "the largest single-year growth of any postcap year" (Lomas *et al*, 1989, p. 93; Hughes 1991, p. 2348).[16] With respect to British Columbia, it is also important to note that fees for physician reimbursements were frozen from 1984 through 1986. However, what is even more important is that in 1983 legislation came into effect requiring new physicians in British Columbia to apply for billing numbers that were "both rationed and geographically restricted (to the less-popular and less-crowded areas)" (Barer *et al*, 1988, p. 34).[17]

In a more recent study on the three provinces of Quebec, Ontario, and British Columbia, between the years 1975 and 1987, it was found that in Quebec utilization per person rose by 68.3%, in Ontario utilization rose by 48.5%, and in British Columbia utilization rose by 45.2% (Hughes 1991, p. 2349). This study, like the previous Canadian study,[18] took into account the fee controls that were in effect in each province during the period studied. These three provinces, which together constitute 74% of Canada's population and 78% of its health care expenditures (Hughes 1991, p. 2347), while they had comparable increases in both population and number of physicians when compared to the United States, had slower rises in physicians' fees.[19] However, "both utilization per person and utilization per physician" increased faster in Canada overall than in the United States (Hughes 1991, p. 2348).

It is studies such as these[20] that have lead Canada's federal Health Minister Benoit Bouchard to conclude that "as many as 30 per cent of medical services performed in Canada do not provide any benefits for patients" (York 1992a, p. A4) and Ontario's Health Minister to warn that the provincial government will "be forced to look at Draconian steps to control the supply of physicians if the medical profession refuses to cooperate" (York 1992b, p. A5) with respect to cost controls, unnecessary services, and geographical distribution. Other provinces in Canada are responding in similar ways. Ontario, for example, recently cut 5,000 hospital jobs, and eliminated 3,500 hospital beds, 2,900 in Toronto alone (Farnsworth 1992, p. 9). In Saskatchewan it was widely feared that the government would reimpose medicare premiums in its recent provincial budget to help offset the province's $517 million deficit for fiscal 1992-93. It did not, but it did cut spending by $344 million and increased taxes by $312 million (Robert 1992, p. A1).

Quebec, which experienced the most phenomenal growth in utilization rates as a response to fee controls, slashed its 1992 health care budget by $270 million per year, and withdraw from its threat to impose "user fees for emergency-room services and massive service cuts" (Picard 1992, p. A5). In British Columbia, they face the "Gretzsky effect," doctors leaving the province for the greener pastures of the United States. For example, the city of Prince George, despite being the third largest city in the province, already suffers from a shortage of doctors. Recent reports indicate that seven more doctors are planning to leave the city to practice in the United States, and 50 more doctors from throughout the province are also considering leaving (B.C. Doctors Looking to Emigrate to the U.S., 1992, p. A4).

British Columbia is also presently facing an additional problem, physicians opting out of the provincial health care plan and billing patients directly for their services. At this time, only 21 of B.C.'s 6,547 physicians have opted out. However, by the end of January 1993, 25 more physicians are expected to join those who have already left. The main reason that doctors are opting out of the province's health care plan is that they are fighting the provincial government's attempt to cap the amount they can earn in a given year, despite the fact that B.C.'s physicians already "have the second highest fee schedule in Canada and earn more for doing less than doctors in most other parts of the country" (Matas 1992, p. A2).

While physicians in both countries may be dissatisfied with their respective fee schedules, health care consumers in both countries are also beginning to manifest their dissatisfaction with their health care providers. The main reasons health care consumers are dissatisfied with their health care systems are as we have argued above: the amount and economic cost of nosocomial infections, iatrogenic injuries, fraud, self-referral, and the practice of physicians inducing demand for their services. In addition to the added economic costs of such practices by the members of the medical profession, health care consumers are not being given the opportunity to consent to these unnecessary diagnostic tests and treatments.

The question of justice in health care arises from within the larger and more complete context of the relationship between providers and consumers of health care. In this chapter we have presented some of the more important evidence concerning the interrelationship between providers and consumers of health care. This evidence, while critical of the meta-structure of health care, is crucial for understanding what justice in health care demands. In the next chapter, we shall offer a comparative analysis of the Canadian and American systems of health care delivery. This analysis, besides identifying the benefits and burdens of each system of health care delivery, will further enlarge the context in which questions of justice in health care are asked and answered.

Chapter II
Canada and the United States:
A Comparative Analysis

Recent polls (Blendon and Taylor, 1989 and Blendon *et al*, 1990. p. 188) have shown that a majority of Americans, 60%, believe that fundamental changes are needed in the U.S. health care system. Another 29% believe that the U.S. health care system should be completely rebuilt, while 10% believe that only minor changes are needed.[21] One need not be all that surprised by the level of dissatisfaction that Americans have with their health care system, for the media are constantly reminding Americans that, not counting the underinsured, there are between 31.1 million (Moyer 1989, p. 104) and 37 million uninsured Americans, or 12.9 to 17.6% of the non-aged population (Brown 1990, p. 413). The highest estimate of the number of uninsured is 48 million (Cangello 1992, p. 31). An intermediate estimate of the number of uninsured is 35.7 million, or 16.6% of Americans (Kalish 1992, p. 8). While estimates of the number of uninsured may vary, it should be noted that all four of the aforementioned authors agree that the majority of uninsured are not the poor but rather the "nonpoor" (Brown 1990, p. 414; Kalish 1992, p. 8; Moyer 1989, p. 105; Cangello 1992, p. 32). The nonpoor, as typically defined by these authors, include those people who are either working or dependents of workers, young adults covered by their parents insurance policy, the self-employed (over 5 million), and part-time workers (Cangello 1992, p. 32). Both

Americans and Canadians are also aware that health care expenditures are consuming an ever increasing percentage of their respective gross national product (GNP). In the United States 12.2% of the GNP or $666.2 billion was spent on health care in 1990. This represents an increase of 10.5% from 1989 (Levit *et al*, 1991b, p. 29), and the largest increase in health care expenditures since 1980 and the second largest increase since 1960 (Levit *et al*, 1991b, p. 30). In Canada in 1988 health care consumed 8.7% of GNP or $50.4 billion ($40.3 billion US) (Rakich 1991b, p. 29). This was an increase of $10.61 billion from the 1985 Canadian health care expenditure figure of $39.79 billion (Crichton *et al*, 1990, p. 28). Moreover, while individual households in the U.S. are spending less of their own personal financial resources for health care in 1990 than they were in 1965, 61% in 1965 versus 35% in 1990, and while business and governments are sharing the ever increasing burden,[22] 29% and 33% respectively (Levit *et al*, 1991a, pp. 83-84), access to health care services is diminishing for an increasing number of Americans.[23]

Further studies suggest that, if current trends continue unabated, U.S. health care expenditures will consume an even larger percentage of the GNP by the year 2000, $1.6 trillion or 16.4% (Sonnefeld *et al*, 1991, p. 1).[24] These and other studies have prompted many in the United States to propose health care reforms.[25] In response many Americans have begun to look north to their neighbor for help in diagnosing and curing the ills of America's health care system.

Compared to Americans, Canadians do seem more satisfied with their health care system. In Canada 38% believe that fundamental charges are needed versus the 60% American figure, 5% believe that the system needs to be completely rebuilt versus the 29% American figure, and 56% believe that only minor changes are needed in Canada's health care system versus the 10% American figure (Blendon *et al*, 1990, p. 188).

The aforementioned expenditure figures, while interesting in and of themselves, do not tell the whole story. While the United States spends 38% more per-capita for health care than Canada, $2,051 versus Canada's $1,483, the United States also spends more per capita for health care than any other OECD (Organization for Economic Cooperation and Development) country (Blendon *et al*, 1990, p. 188; Southby and Rakich, 1991, p. 11). Furthermore, while health care expenditures as a percentage of gross domestic product (GDP)[26] have increased much more rapidly in the United States than in Canada since 1960, 5.5% in Canada in 1960 to 8.8% in Canada in 1987 versus 5.2% in the U.S. in 1960 to 11.2% in the U.S. in 1987 (Schieber 1990, p. 159; Pfaff 1990, p. 3), the United States continues to rank lower in terms of life expectancy and infant survival rate. Life expectancy for both Canadian men, 73.1 years, and women, 79.9 years, in 1986 was greater than that for American men, 71.3 years, and women, 78.3 years (General Accounting Office 1991, p. 16).[27] Canadians also fared better with respect to infant mortality rates. In Canada in 1987 the infant mortality rate was 7.3 deaths per 1,000 live births versus the U.S. rate of 10.1 deaths per 1,000 live births (General Accounting Office, 1991. p. 16).[28]

Some have argued that because of Canada's (alleged) success at controlling health care costs (Barer and Evans, 1992; Evans *et al*, 1989; Barer and Evans, 1986; Pfaff, 1990), or because of socio-cultural parallels that currently exist between Canada and the United States (Sakala 1990), or because a free market[29] in health care insurance is not possible (Enthoven 1988), or because of the U.S.'s (alleged) failure at controlling its "overhead component of health insurance" (Evans *et al*, 1989, p. 572),[30] or because of the U.S.'s alleged failure to control administrative costs[31] that Canada's universal health care system, or at least aspects of it (Blendon *et al*, 1992), is the model best suited to meet American's health care needs.[32] Most recently the U.S. General Accounting Office concluded, on the basis of these earlier estimates, that

if the United States were to shift to a system of universal coverage and a single payer, as in Canada, the savings in administrative costs would be more than enough to offset the expense of universal coverage (General Accounting Office 1991, pp. 6-7).

Critics, in response, have been quick to point out that Canada's health care system is not without its difficulties and that the U.S. will be better served if it does not adopt a Canadian model of health care delivery (Danzon 1992; Goodman and Musgrave, 1991; Haislmaier 1991; Kosterlitz 1989a and 1989b; Lindsay *et al*, 1978; Neuschler 1990; Rakich 1991a and 1991b; Swartz 1991; Van Loon 1986; Walker 1989 and 1992; Mitchell 1988).

Given this divergence of opinion on the merits and demerits of the Canadian system of health care delivery, in order to assess it as a possible system of health care delivery for the United

States, we need to know more about its evolution, its strengths, its weaknesses, and how it differs from the system of health care delivery in the United States. Hence, in what immediately follows we describe the four key pieces of federal legislation responsible for the evolution of Canada's health care system. We then present a brief overview of the American health care system, followed by an overview of some of the more pressing concerns of an increasing number of health care consumers in both countries.

Canadians, through their tax system, share both the risk and cost of disease and injury through their national health care system. The genesis[33] of the existing system of health care delivery in Canada began in the province of Saskatchewan in 1946 when the Saskatchewan provincial government, which was then ruled by the Commonwealth Cooperative Federation party, introduced a government sponsored hospital insurance program.[34] The principle component of this program was that "hospital coverage was to be universal and comprehensive in that all essential services within reasonable limits should be provided and that there would be no limit on the number of days of hospitalization that would be covered" (Abelson 1992, p. 5). The money to pay for the program was to be collected in the form of a premium from those who could afford to pay. In the late 1940s both British Columbia and Alberta adopted similar hospital insurance programs (Abelson 1992, p. 5; Crichton *et al*, 1990, p. 164).

In 1957, the federal government of Canada, which was a liberal government at the time, in a unanimous decision passed the Hospitals Insurance and Diagnostic Act. It was this Act which gave Canadians its first health insurance program that was supported at the national level (Crichton *et al*, 1990, pp. 191-196). The effect of this legislation was to introduce interprovincial cost-sharing for the operating expenses of hospitals. However, it was not until 1961, when Quebec joined, that all ten provinces and the two territories participated in the system. In order to participate each province's hospital insurance plan had meet the following conditions: the plan had to be "universally available to provincial residents, be portable, assure adequate hospital standards, assure that adequate records and accounts were kept, and ensure public administration" (Crichton *et al*, 1990, p. 32). The cost sharing arrangement of this act provided for the federal government to pay

25% of national per capita costs and 25% of provincial per capita costs. This figure was then multiplied by the number of insured persons. The participating provinces were then responsible for the remainder of their costs (Crichton *et al*, 1990, p. 34; Rakich 1991a, p. 15). The conditions for participation in this cost-sharing arrangement were the precursor to the conditions of the next important piece of legislation, the Medical Care Act of 1966 (Crichton *et al*, 1990, pp. 32-35; Abelson 1992, pp. 8-10; Lindsay *et al*, 1978, p. 5).

The Medical Care Act was passed by a virtually unanimous vote on July 1, 1966 -- which, by the way, is Canada Day. This Act, which is without a doubt the most important Act in the history of Canada's system of health care delivery, covered physician services and specified four of the five determining principles of Canada's present health care delivery system: universality, comprehensiveness, portability, and public administration (Crichton *et al*, 1990, pp. 32-35; Abelson 1992, pp. 8-10; Lindsay *et al*, 1978, p. 5; Sakala 1990, pp. 716-717). The principal effect of the Medical Care Act was that the federal and provincial governments would split the cost for medical fees if the provincial governments agreed to the four principles; the federal government would pay 50% of each province's cost and each province would pay the remaining 50%. The four principles were defined as follows:

1. comprehensiveness, that is, coverage of all insured health services provided by hospitals, medical practitioners or dentists and others where permitted;
2. universality, that is, 100 percent of insured persons were to be entitled to insured health services under uniform terms and conditions, with a waiting period for provincial residents not to exceed three months;
3. portability, that is, residents moving to another province would be covered during the waiting period by the old province;
4. public administration by a public nonprofit authority responsible to the provincial government, subject to audit (Crichton *et al*, 1990, p. 33).

The Medical Care Act took effect in July 1968, and by April 1971, the Northwest Territories joined making the Medical Care Act the rule of the land.

The following encapsulates the entry dates for each province and territory into the Hospitals Insurance and Diagnostic Act

(HIDS) and the Medical Care Act (MCA) (Lindsay *et al*, 1978, p. 6):

Province	HIDS	MCA
Newfoundland	7/1/58	4/1/69
Prince Edward Island	10/1/59	12/1/70
Nova Scotia	1/1/59	4/1/69
New Brunswick	7/1/59	1/1/71
Quebec	1/1/61	11/1/70
Ontario	1/1/59	10/1/69
Manitoba	7/1/58	4/1/69
Alberta	7/1/58	7/1/69
British Columbia	7/1/58	7/1/68
Yukon	7/1/60	4/1/72
Northwest Territories	4/1/60	4/1/71

In 1977, in an attempt to reduce federal health care expenditures (Crichton *et al*, 1990, p. 33; Abelson 1992, pp. 10-12), the federal government enacted the Established Programs Financing Act (EPF).[35] This Act repealed both the Hospitals Insurance and Diagnostic Act and the Medical Care Act, as well as the provisions for post-secondary education,[36] and it reconstituted the federal-provincial cost-sharing arrangement. Under the new arrangement of Established Programs Financing Act the federal government was to give each province an annual amount linked to population, changes in the GNP, and a federal tax transfer to each of the provinces and the two territories. In addition, the poorer provinces, typically the Atlantic provinces, were to be given equalization payments (Crichton *et al*, 1990, p. 34, and pp. 197-208; Abelson 1992, p. 11).

The new cost-sharing arrangement of the Established Programs Financing Act meant that the federal government had less influence on how each province administered its health care budget. It also meant that the provinces, rather than the federal government, had to suffer the political consequences of cost-control measures (Crichton *et al*, 1990, pp. 34-35; Rakich 1991a, p. 15). Another effect of the Established Programs Financing Act was that the provinces, in order to increase revenues, turned to user fees, while allowing physicians the practice of extra-billing. The Canadian practice of extra-billing is comparable to the American practice of balance billing (Rakich 1991b, p. 27).[37] These practices, which the federal government feared would compromise universality, led Federal Health Minister Monique Bégin to pass the Canada Health Act in 1984.

The stated purpose of the Canada Health Act was "to establish criteria and conditions that must be met before full payment may be made under the Act of 1977 [that is, the Established Programs Financing Act] in respect of insured health services and extended health services provided under provincial law" (Crichton *et al*, 1990, p. 35). The five criteria, four of which were previously established under the Medical Care Act, were universality, comprehensiveness, portability, public administration, and accessibility. This latter condition was defined as "reasonable access by insured persons to insured health services unprecluded or unimpeded, either directly or indirectly, by charges or other means" (Crichton *et al*, 1990, p. 35). In effect this meant that provinces would have to legislate away the practices of extra-billing and user fees. After three years of fierce federal-provincial political battles, and the Ontario doctor's strike[38] in June of 1986, all provinces accepted the provisions of the Canada Health Act in 1987.[39]

Funding of the 1,230 hospitals[40] in Canada is primarily the responsibility of provincial governments, although they do receive federal funds from cost-sharing. Provincial ministers of health are given a budget which they then proceed to distribute negotiated amounts to the hospitals under their jurisdiction. Canada's hospital administrators are responsible for operating their hospital within the confines of the budget they receive, delivering care to all who enter their doors.

Most hospitals in Canada were constructed between 1948 and 1980, with a gradual slowing from 1970 onward due to cost control (Crichton *et al*, 1990, p. 82). In Canada hospitals are typically nonprofit corporate entities, although there are provincial variations. Hospitals are governed by provincial legislation, which usually requires hospital board members to draft bylaws for their operation. With respect to physicians, Canadian doctors for the most part, like their American counterparts, are paid on a fee-for-service basis.[41]

Canada does not have one single health care plan but rather twelve, that is one for each of the ten provinces and two territories. Yet notwithstanding the number of health care plans in the country Canadian citizens, like their American counterparts, are free to choose their own physician. However, unlike their American counterparts, Canadians have, at the point of consumption, virtually free access to health care. The minor exception to this generalization is that residents of both Alberta and British Columbia are charged a nominal premium for their health care insurance, however, because the premiums are not based on risk they are in effect taxes (Rakich 1991a, p. 17). The remainder of Canadian health care expenditures for covered health care expenses comes from public sources.[42] It is this public financing of health care in Canada that is ultimately responsible for the universal and comprehensive coverage enjoyed by (approximately) 25 million Canadians. It is also the method of financing health care that distinguishes Canada's health care delivery system from its American counterpart.

In the United States, with the exception of Medicaid which is state funded and Medicare[43] which is federally funded, health care is privately financed via a multitude of insurance companies, or as they are often referred to, third-party payers. This method of financing health care has profound implications with respect to access to health care in the United States; 31 to 37 million Americans are uninsured. That is, there are more uninsured Americans than the entire population of Canada.[44] In the United States "180 million residents have privately financed health insurance, with 82 percent receiving it from employers" (Rakich 1991b, p. 27). The range of this coverage varies from minimum to full depending on the particular policy one purchases.

If one compares Canada to the United States, with the exception of size and the percentage of population over age 65, one should think, roughly, in terms of tenths.[45] Canada's population in 1986 was 25.3 million, versus a U.S. population of 241.6 million. Using U.S dollars, the GNP of Canada in 1987 was $394.4 billion versus $4,526.7 billion in the United States; Canada's federal budget in fiscal year 1986/87 was $116.4 billion versus the U.S. federal budget of $1,004.6 billion. In 1988 Canada spent a total of $50.4 billion on health care expenditures versus the U.S.'s $496.6 billion, or, respectively, 8.7% and 11.2% of GNP. In Canada per capita health care expenditures amounted to $1,556 versus $1,973 in the United States in 1988.

Some important non-monetary figures are the (1985) number of physicians, 52,000 versus the U.S.'s 577,000; the ratio of physicians to population in 1985 was 486 compared to the U.S.'s

418; the total number of all hospitals in Canada in 1987 numbered 1,218 versus the U.S.'s 6,841; and the total number of beds for each country was 178,565 versus the U.S.'s 1,290,000. This calculates out to a beds per thousand ratio of 7.1 and 5.4 respectively. Canada's hospital occupancy rate in 1987 was somewhat higher than the U.S. rate, 83.8% versus 68.4% respectively. The number of full-time equivalent hospital employees in the same year was 393,000 versus the U.S.'s 3,647,000. This leads to a full-time equivalent (hospital employee) per bed ratio of 2.2 versus the U.S.'s 2.8. In Canada, in 1987, expenditures for physician services consumed 15.7% of health care expenditures, while in the United States physician services consumed 19.6% of American health care expenditures. Hospital expenditures in 1987 accounted for 40% of the total of Canadian health care expenditures, while in the United States hospital expenditures accounted for 39.6% of American health care expenditures.

The United States leads Canada in both high-tech equipment and procedures, even when comparing 1987 U.S. figures with Canada's 1989 figures.[46] The reason for this American lead in high-tech equipment and procedures may be, as Weisbrod argues, that in the United States research and development of high-tech medical equipment and procedures shares a reciprocal relationship with the expected utilization of the results of research and development and the demand for health care insurance. This may explain, at least in part, the U.S.'s role as leader in the field of high-tech medicine (Weisbrod 1991). The United States has 900 MRI units compared to Canada's 12; 228 lithotripsy units (a device used to break up kidney stones) to Canada's 4; and 967 radiotherapy units to Canada's 14. Furthermore, the United States has 793 open-heart surgery units compared to Canada's 32; 1,234 cardia catheterization units to Canada's 39, and 319 organ transplant units compared to Canada's 28 units (Rublee 1989, p. 180).

There are other substantial social, economic, political, legal, and demographic differences between Canada and the United States, some of which are outlined below. For our immediate purposes, however, the most significant difference is political. Americans have a much stronger individualist ethic than Canadians and they also distrust their government more than most Canadians. This difference would play an important role if the United States, as the General Accounting Office report and others have argued for, adopted a Canadian-style system of health care. However, given the current political climate in the United States, the United States is not likely to adopt a Canadian-style health care system, especially in the light of three recent studies that challenge the earlier findings on saving administrative costs by adopting a Canadian-style system.[47]

The first study criticizes the particular method used to calculate the earlier estimates, a "simple comparison of accounting costs" (Danzon 1992, p. 40). Danzon also criticizes the earlier studies for their failure to include the hidden costs of the Canadian health care system. For example, she argues that earlier studies failed to include "excessive patient time costs that result from the proliferation of multiple short visits in response to controls on physicians' fee; diminished productivity and quality of life from delay or unavailability of surgical procedures, and loss of productivity due to underuse of some medical procedures" (Danzon 1992, pp. 30-31), and the "hidden costs of tax-based financing" (Danzon 1992, pp. 36-37). She concludes that "the rough empirical evidence tends to confirm that overhead costs in Canada, adjusted to include some of the most significant hidden costs, are indeed higher than they are under private insurance in the United States" (Danzon 1992, p. 40).

The second study focused on the increased utilization the United States health care system would experience if it adopted a Canadian model of health care. The study criticizes the earlier studies for failing to include "many of the overhead costs associated with administering the program in Canada, such as buildings, equipment, fringe benefits, and personnel services" (Shiels *et al*, 1992, p. 11). The authors of this study estimate that the United States would indeed save administrative costs from adopting a model of the Canadian health care system; "overall, nationwide insurer administrative costs would be reduced from $38.2 billion under current policy to $15.7 billion under the Canadian model, for a net savings of $22.5 billion" (Shiels *et al*, 1992, p. 12). With respect to physician administrative costs, the authors concede that a Canadian model would reduce such costs by $11 billion in 1991 (Shiels *et al*, 1992, p. 14). This amount would be achieved by duplicating Canada's monopsonist policy, by using a standard "electronic claims-filing process," and eliminating "many of the prospective utilization management programs" (Shiels *et al*, 1992, p. 13). In addition they estimate, for various reasons (Shiels *et al*,

1992, pp. 14-16), that hospital administrative costs could also be reduced to the tune of some $13.5 billion (Shiels *et al*, 1992, p. 160). However, they subsequently go on to estimate that "increased utilization by previously uninsured persons could raise costs by $11.1 billion" (Shiels *et al*, 1992, p. 16), that eliminating cost sharing would cost another $49.7 billion (Shiels *et al*, 1992, p. 16), that increased utilization of nursing homes and home health services would cost an additional $10.2 billion (Shiels *et al*, 1992, p. 17). Thus when all the adding and subtracting is completed, they conclude "the increase in utilization under the Canadian model ($78.2 billion) would exceed administrative savings ($46.9 billion) by $31.4 billion" (Shiels *et al*, 1992, p. 20).

It should be noted that neither of these two studies, nor the earlier studies which estimated savings in administrative costs, took into consideration several other important factors, such as the substantially higher number of veterans in the United States as compared to Canada, the substantially higher rate of violent crime,[48] homicide[49] (especially for young black males),[50] drug abuse, AIDS,[51] the divorce rate,[52] drug exposed babies,[53] and other socio-demographic factors. If one adds just together the costs of the U.S.'s social ills, they exceed by far the total amount of Canada's national health care expenditures. Canada also lags substantially behind the United States when it comes to several important medical technologies and procedures, as outlined earlier.

In addition, the United States has a history of being a much more highly litigious society than Canada. However, when it comes to medical malpractice, the differences are not as pronounced as one might have expected. "The rate of growth of malpractice claim frequency and severity has been as high in Canada and the United Kingdom over the last two decades as in the United States, although levels remain higher in the United States" (Danzon 1991, p. 58). There is good evidence (as we documented in the previous chapter) for the existence of medical malpractice in both countries for, as some have phrased it, "medical care is a risky business" (Weiler *et al*, 1992, p. 2355), especially for the health care consumer.

We have compared Canada's universal health care system with that of the United States. In the course of this comparative analysis, we discovered, among other things, that while Canada may spend less per capita on health care than the United States, it has its own unique set of problems. These ranged from substantially less high-tech equipment and procedures per capita than the United States. In addition, Canadians suffer other costs, from lengthy waits for some surgeries to having to leave the country in order to obtain other surgeries. Canada's hospital facilities are also older than their U.S counterparts.

Both countries face escalating costs for health care services, despite efforts in both countries to control costs. The empirical evidence suggests that physicians in both countries induce demand for their services when threatened with cost-containment measures. It is important to realize that the cost of this induced demand should not just be measured in monetary costs; one also needs to bear in mind that people incur various minor iatrogenic injuries from these excess medical services, not to mention severe disabilities and/or death. In addition, as we also mentioned, the practice of induced demand by physicians precludes their obtaining an informed consent from their patient.

It is the larger context of health care, including both its benefits and deficiencies, that a theory of justice in health care must contend with. We have not focused on the particular benefits clinical medicine, as opposed to the institution of medicine, has to offer. Our reasons for this was that these benefits are more well known than the deficiencies and therefore the emphasis was well placed. With the larger context of medical care before us, we now turn to consider two alternative theories of justice in health care.

Chapter III
Fair Equality of Opportunity and Justice in Health Care

In the previous chapters, in addition to giving an overview of both the Canadian and the American health care delivery systems, we identified some issues that are of concern to both consumers and providers of health care. The more important of the issues identified were the number of underinsured and uninsured, the problem of self-referral by physicians, the problem of induced demand, unnecessary and inappropriate care, iatrogenic injuries, and nosocomial infections. We suggested, directly and indirectly, that it is within this broader context that discussions of rights to health care need to take place. In this and the next chapter, we narrow the scope of our investigation to consider two alternative approaches that have been used to support a view of justice in health care, that of Norman Daniels and Allen Buchanan.

While the approaches taken by Daniels and Buchanan may differ substantially in form, content, and conclusions, they do share a certain similarity. Both are concerned to defend a right to health care, albeit they differ in the form that might take. In Daniels' case not only does he attempt to defend a positive right to health care, he also attempts to defend a comprehensive theory of justice in health care based on an amended version of John Rawls' principle of fair equality of opportunity (Rawls 1971). Buchanan, on the other hand, attempts to defend just a positive right to a decent minimum of health care and principally on the strength of what he terms his two enforced beneficence arguments. The arguments by Buchanan and Daniels can be viewed as complementing each other, especially when Daniels admits that not all persons will fall under the umbrella of his fair equality of opportunity argument and that "principles of beneficence may be an important guide to our obligations" (Daniels 1985, p. 48). Buchanan's enforced beneficence arguments may provide the needed support for Daniels argument's weakness. By saying this I do not mean to suggest that they were written for that purpose. All I mean to suggest is that Buchanan's argument might provide needed support for one of the admitted weaknesses in Daniels' approach.

Both contributions, however, are important. In Daniels' case, the importance lies not only in his attempt to extend Rawls' principle of fair equality of opportunity to cover a positive right to health care, but also in a number of other important health care related issues, from a reason for thinking that health care is a special social good to addressing the problem of access to health care and the problem of distributing health-care resources between the young and old.[54] He also uses his theory to address a number of other important issues, such as possible interference with the health care provider's autonomy, preventive health care, and health-hazard regulation in the workplace. Buchanan's contribution, although not as comprehensive as Daniels', in addition to defending a positive right to a "decent"[55] minimum of health care and offering an important new approach for resolving certain kinds of public policy issues, can also be viewed as an attempt to establish a positive right to health care for those who are not covered under Daniels' umbrella. If both or either arguments are successful, then one of the more troubling issues in biomedical ethics will have been resolved. However, we shall argue that they are unsuccessful and that another approach might succeed where they have failed.

We begin with a brief explication of Daniels' fair equality of opportunity argument, illustrating its conceptual connection to its Rawlsian predecessor. However, given that our main concern is Daniels and not Rawls, we need not enter the debate over which of the many interpretations is the best interpretation of Rawls' view.[56] For our purposes it is sufficient if we merely briefly explicate Rawls' argument for the principles of justice and elucidate the relationship between Daniels' use of the Rawlsian principle of fair equality of opportunity and Rawls' general theory of distributive justice.

Rawls' principal concern was to identify principles of justice. In support of this end he placed hypothetical people, who were conceived to be free, equal, and mutually disinterested, behind a "veil of ignorance." Rawls conceived the people behind the veil of ignorance to be people who do not take "an interest in one another's interests" (Rawls 1971, p. 13); that is, they were to recognize each other as potential partners in "a cooperative venture for mutual advantage" (Rawls 1971, p. 4). The principles chosen from behind the veil of ignorance are to govern the distribution of primary social goods, where primary social goods are defined as those things that every rational person is presumed to want, whatever else he might want (Rawls 1971, p. 62).

Rawls characterizes the people behind the veil of ignorance -- given their situation and what is at stake -- as extremely cautious, and argues that they would employ the maximin rule in making their decision. That is, the people are to "rank alternatives by their worst possible outcomes" and then "adopt the alternative the worst outcome of which is superior to the worst outcomes of the others" (Rawls 1971, pp. 152-53). Rawls argues that the people in the original position would choose two principles of justice: the equal liberty principle, and the difference principle. He also argues that these principles are lexically ordered (Rawls 1971, pp. 42-45). To say that these principles are lexically ordered is to say that we are to satisfy all requirements of the first principle prior to satisfying the requirements of the later principles.

The equal liberty principle simply states that each person should have an equal right to the most extensive system of equal basic liberty compatible with a similar system of liberty for all. The difference principle is composed of two parts. It says that "social and economic inequalities are to be arranged so that they are both (a) to the greatest benefit of the least advantaged, consistent with the just savings principle, and (b) attached to offices and positions open to all under conditions of fair equality of opportunity" (Rawls 1971, p. 302).

Daniels attempts to argue for a positive right to health care by extending the Rawlsian principle of fair equality of opportunity so that health care institutions would be included among the basic institutions that a society commits to ensuring fair equality of opportunity. His argument for this has three stages. First, he argues that health care is a "special social good" (Daniels 1985, p. 56) because of its limited role in maintaining species-typical normal functioning. He then argues that impairment of species-typical normal functioning has an adverse impact on one's normal opportunity range, where a normal opportunity range is defined as "the array of life plans reasonable persons in [a society] are likely to construct for themselves" (Daniels 1985, p. 33). Second, because disease and illness are like lack of talent and/or skill in that they adversely affect the range of opportunities one may have in a modern liberal democratic society, he argues, one should not be denied access to the full scope of one's normal opportunity range simply on the basis of the "natural disadvantages induced by disease" (Daniels 1985, p. 46). Finally, assuming that justice requires guaranteeing fair equality of opportunity, then, Daniels concludes, health-care institutions should be among those basic institutions which are governed by a principle that will guarantee fair equality of opportunity. He says:

> I urge the fair equality of opportunity principle as an appropriate principle to govern macro decisions about the design of our health-care system. Such a principle defines, from the perspective of justice, what the moral function of the health-care system must be - to help guarantee fair equality of opportunity. This is the fundamental insight underlying the approach developed here (Daniels 1985, p. 41).

Daniels buttresses the first stage of his argument for basing a positive right to health care on his Rawlsian-like principle of fair equality of opportunity with the argument that in order to generate the conclusion that health care is a special social good we need a theory of health-care needs. Health-care needs, he tells us, are "those things we need in order to maintain, restore, or provide functional equivalents (where possible) to normal species functioning" (Daniels 1985, p. 32). The theory of health-care needs on which Daniels relies is Christopher Boorse's biomedical model (Boorse 1981). Daniels-cum-Boorse's account of the biomedical model of health-care needs is that "health is the absence of disease, and diseases (I include deformities and disabilities that result from trauma) are deviations from the natural functional organization of a typical member of a species"

(Daniels 1985, p. 28). The list of needs Daniels includes under health-care needs is substantial. He includes all of the following (Daniels 1985, p. 32):

1. Adequate nutrition, shelter
2. Sanitary, safe, unpolluted living and working conditions
3. Exercise, rest, and some other features of lifestyle
4. Preventive, curative, and rehabilitative personal medical services
5. Non-medical personal and social support services

These health-care needs can be met, Daniels argues, by a four-tier system of health-care delivery.

The primary function of the first tier, preventive health care services, would be to avert deviations from species-typical normal functioning. The primary function of the second tier, personal medical and rehabilitative services, would be to correct deviations from species-typical normal functioning. The third tier, extended and chronic medical care and social support services, would provide the necessary services to those whose medical conditions were such that, while they could not be cured, they could be either maintained at their current level of functioning and/or prevented from deteriorating further. Finally, the fourth tier, palliative care institutions, would serve those whose medical conditions were beyond the ken and machinations of medical technology such that they cannot be "brought closer to the idealization" (Daniels 1985, pp. 47-48) of species-typical normal functioning.

It is here we note the potential conceptual connection between Daniels' fair equality of opportunity argument and Buchanan's enforced beneficence arguments. Daniels concedes that with respect to this fourth tier of health care delivery services we may be "beyond measures that justice requires" (Daniels 1985, p. 48). If there are certain people for whom there is no chance of protecting opportunity then, according to Daniels' fair equality of opportunity argument, they may not be entitled to any health care services. Daniels readily admits this and simply claims that "principles of beneficence may be an important guide to our obligations" (Daniels 1985, p. 48). Buchanan's arguments for enforced beneficence, although not intentionally written as a support for this admitted weakness, may provide the support that Daniels was unable to muster in this regard. We shall return to this matter in Chapter IV.

While Daniels' fair equality of opportunity argument does not guarantee a universal individual positive right[57] to health care, it would guarantee that we would have those "rights and entitlements [that are] defined within a set of basic institutions governed by the fair equality of opportunity principle" (Daniels 1985, p. 54). These basic institutions -- essentially the four-tier health care delivery system outlined above, or to be more precise, the first three tiers -- are, on Daniels' account, necessary to provide what a theory of justice in health care requires if our general theory of distributive justice guarantees that we are to have fair equality of opportunity.

While Daniels' argument may be related to Rawls' argument there are important differences, especially concerning the fair equality of opportunity principle. On Rawls' account the fair equality of opportunity principle is, first and foremost, argued for. It is, Rawls argues, a principle of distributive justice that would be chosen by free, rational, equal, and mutually disinterested agents behind a veil of ignorance. On Daniels' account the fair equality of opportunity principle is assumed at the outset. Thus it is worth noting that, in fact, Daniels' argument is a conditional argument. He says:

> In this book I have argued that, if it is a requirement of justice that basic social institutions guarantee fair equality of opportunity, then health-care institutions should be among those regulated by the equal opportunity principle (Daniels 1985, p. 117).

That Daniels' fair equality of opportunity argument is a conditional argument is important for at least two reasons. The first reason is that alternative theories of justice -- for example, Nozick's entitlement theory of justice (Nozick 1974), Gauthier's hypothetical contractarianism (Gauthier 1986) and utilitarian theories of justice -- may not include a principle of justice which requires our basic social institutions to guarantee fair equality of opportunity. The second reason for noting the structure of Daniels' argument is that the antecedent of the conditional, his appeal to, as well as his reliance on, fair equality of opportunity as a principle of distributive justice, is deeply problematic. We shall return to the issue of alternative theories of justice in the following chapter when we consider Buchanan's enforced beneficence argument for a positive right to a decent minimum of health care. In later chapters we employ Gauthier's theory of justice in arguing for a positive right to a just minimum of health care. The problems associated with Daniels' use of the Rawlsian principle of fair equality of opportunity will be dealt with after we consider a second importance difference between Rawls' and Daniels' account of fair equality of opportunity.

The second difference between Rawls' and Daniels' account of fair equality of opportunity is that the scope of opportunity Rawls had in mind is much narrower than the scope Daniels has in mind. Rawls' conception of fair equality of opportunity relates to the likelihood one has in a just society of securing one of the better positions that society has to offer. Daniels' conception of fair equality of opportunity is much broader in the sense that it relates to the likelihood one has in a just society of actualizing any one of the "array of life plans reasonable persons are likely to construct for themselves" (Daniels 1985, p. 33). Given that Daniels' conception of fair equality of opportunity is much broader than Rawls', then, as Stern notes and Buchanan reiterates (Buchanan 1984, pp. 63-64), "Daniels' FEO [Fair Equality of Opportunity] requires promoting equality in more areas of life than Rawlsian FEO" (Stern 1983, p. 340).[58] The promotion of equality in more areas of life is problematic for, if it cannot be constrained, society may find itself attempting to meet all health care needs in the name of fair equality of opportunity. Any such attempt would place us on the edge of a "bottomless pit" (Fried 1978, chap. 5; Daniels 1985, p. 53) that has the potential to consume not only our health care budget but all of society's resources.

As noted in Chapter I, the bottomless pit problem is that there is potentially an unlimited need for the benefits medical technology makes possible, but there are limits on the amount of resources that a society can commit to health care. For example, as we noted in the previous chapter, the U.S.'s 1990 health care expenditures were 12.2% of the GNP or $666.2 billion (Levit *et al*, 1991b, p. 29). They are projected to increase to $1.6 trillion, or 16.4 % by the turn of the century (Sonnefeld *et al*, 1991, p. 1). As we also noted in the previous chapter, this projected amount would be more than the current cost of "education, defense, and recreation combined" (Smith 1991, p. 44). Consequently, given the amount that could be spent on health care, the cost of health care consumption needs to be constrained. Various measures to control costs have been imposed on both sides of the border but with limited success in both Canada and the United States due to the problem of physicians inducing demand for their services (Rakich and Becker, 1992; Fuchs and Hahn, 1990; Contandriopoulos 1986).

Two versions of the bottomless pit problem can be distinguished, the theory-independent and the theory-dependent version. In the first version, the theory-independent version, there exists the theoretical potential that health care could consume most of a society's resources. For example and as noted above, U.S. health care expenditures are projected to consume 16.4% of the American GNP by the end of this decade. If the U.S. does not curtail the rate of increase in consumption of health care, then this figure could continue to rise to even an even higher percentage of the American GNP. In the theory-dependent version of the bottomless pit problem, there still exists the potential for health care expenditures to consume the majority of a society's resources but in this case the potential is limited by the theory in terms of what health care consumption is allowed. For example, a theory of justice in health care, in order to avoid the theory-dependent version of the bottomless pit problem, must offer some device from within the theory to constrain the cost of health care consumption, such that a given health care budget will meet the needs implied by the theory. In what follows, we shall only be concerned with the theory-dependent version of the bottomless pit problem. We shall argue that Daniels' theory of justice in health care fails for the reason that it fails to provide a device from within his theory that will disarm the threat posed by the theory-dependent version of the bottomless pit problem.

There are three considerations that any theory of justice in health care must account for in resolving the theory-dependent version of the bottomless pit problem (Wikler 1983, pp. 119-120). The first consideration is the theory's scope of application, or the range of people assumed to be covered under the theory. The second consideration that any theory of justice in health care must account for is the supply of people who are sick and/or injured. This supply is virtually inexhaustible. Not only does our progeny ensure an inexhaustible supply, but also as people move through life's various stages they encounter various diseases, accidents, and/or injuries, thus compounding the problem of supply. Some of these conditions may be trivial. Others however, and this accents the difficulty posed by the first consideration, are exceptional in the amount of health care resources they threaten to consume. The third consideration that a theory of justice in health care must deal with in order to resolve the bottomless pit problem is ensuring that the benefits of medical treatments and/or diagnostic procedures outweigh the costs of such treatments and/or procedures. In addition to addressing, in turn, each of these considerations more fully in what follows, we shall argue that the main reason Daniels' theory of justice in health care cannot resolve the theory-dependent version of the bottomless pit problem is that there is nothing within the theory that can either circumvent or mitigate the three considerations identified above.

In any society there exists some percentage of the population that is the most sick and/or injured. In many cases, this group of people will simply fall outside of the scope of the theory in question. For example, Daniels has conceded that if there are people who are so sick and/or injured that they cannot benefit in terms of protecting and/or maintaining their access to their normal opportunity range, then they are simply beyond the scope of his theory of just health care. However, even if there exists a group of people who are outside of the scope of a theory's range of application, there will always exist another group of the most sick and/or injured who do fall within the bounds covered by the theory, the next most sick and/or injured. Therefore we distinguish the restricted version of this problem from the unrestricted version. The restricted version of this problem, as it applies to Daniels' theory, will encompass those of the most sick and injured who can benefit in terms of improving and/or protecting their normal opportunity range, while the unrestricted version of this problem will encompass those of the most sick and injured who cannot benefit in terms of improving and/or protecting their normal opportunity range and who are, therefore, beyond the scope of his theory. We shall only concern ourselves with the restricted version of this problem and we will refer to this problem as the morbidity problem.

In a recent study of Ohio's Blue Cross-Blue Shield benefit payments, for example, it was found that of all those insured, 90% received benefit payments averaging only $794. The remaining 10%, who had major health problems, averaged $10,529. Thus 10% of beneficiaries accounted for almost $79.7 million of the $123 million paid out, or 65%. Furthermore, of that 10%, 1% received $29.1 million, or 37% of the $79.7 million. Overall this 1% accounted for 24% of the $123 million paid (Wicker 1991, p. A7). If this pattern held roughly true across the board, which isn't an unrealistic assumption given that "only 11.5% of the population is hospitalized each year" and of that 11.5% that is hospitalized 15% "account for more than half (55%) of hospital expenditures" (Gagner 1992c, p. 26), then by simple extrapolation of the latest American health care expenditures, this would mean that of the $666.2 billion spent on health care in 1990 (Levit *et al*, 1991b, p. 29) $433.03 billion of health care expenditures would have been consumed by 10% of the population; that is $10.43 billion more than the $422.6 billion (Levit *et al*, 1991b, p. 46) spent on health care in 1985. Of that $433.03 billion, 1% of the population would have consumed $160.22 billion; that is $27.32 billion more than the $132.9 billion (Lazenby and Letsch, 1990, p. 14) spent on health care in 1975. Of the total 1990 health care expenditure of $666.2 billion, that 1% of the population would have consumed $159.89 billion; that is $26.99 billion more than the total 1975 expenditure of $132.9 billion.[59]

If this trend held true for the future, then, looking at projected health care expenditures for 1992 where national health care expenditures are expected to reach $809 billion, or 14.7% of that year's GNP (Sonnefeld *et al*, 1991, p. 1), we would find that just 10% of the population would consume $525.85 billion by the end of this year, or $31.75 billion less than the total 1987 expenditure of $494.1 billion (Levit *et al*, 1991b, p. 47). And further, 1% of that 10% would, by the end of this year, consume $194.56 billion, or $61.66 billion more than the $132.9 billion spent in 1975.

Daniels has conceded that if health care cannot benefit someone with respect to their opportunity range, then it is not a requirement of justice that they be given health care but rather they can only rely on their own resources or the beneficence of their fellow man. If we assume that only the top 1% of the 10% of the population that is the most ill is such that health care will not benefit them with respect to their opportunity range, then, for 1992 alone, we could reap savings of $194.56 billion. However, that would still leave us with 9% of the population consuming $331.29 billion in 1992 alone. This is still $82.19 billion more than the $249.1 billion (Lazenby and Letsch, 1990, p. 14) that was spent on health care in 1980.

If we look at the morbidity problem from another angle, similar results obtain. It has been noted that 14%, or "one in every seven health care dollars being spent each year is on the last six months of someone's life" (Clark 1992, p. 19). Thus in 1990, the year in which the most recent figures are available, that would amount to $93.27 billion of the $666.2 billion spent that year going to people in the last six months of their life. Of course, it is difficult to speculate what portion of that $93.27 billion could be saved by not treating those of the assumed 1% of the population who, on Daniels' account, would not have a claim on health care resources because there would be no positive effect on their opportunity range. But nonetheless, the point remains: we don't always know what the outcome of medical treatment will be[60] and so if there is a chance that treating someone will have a positive effect on their opportunity range, then, on Daniels' account, we must treat them, even though they may die within six months. If Daniels cannot find the means to constrain health care consumption, then it is possible that less than 10% of the population could consume most of the available health care resources.

The second consideration that any theory of justice in health care must deal with is the sheer number of people who could benefit from medical treatment in terms of maintaining and/or improving their access to their normal opportunity range; the supply of both the sick and injured, as noted earlier, is virtually inexhaustible. The problem posed by the supply of people who could benefit in terms of maintaining and/or improving their access to their normal opportunity range is not simply the same difficulty posed by the morbidity problem. The difficulty the supply problem poses, unlike the morbidity problem, does not have to do with the severity of certain diseases and/or injuries, but rather it has to do with the number of people who are so afflicted. In the United States, for example, between 1972 and 1981 the number of people requiring coronary bypass surgery and hip arthroplasties (total hip replacement), have both increased dramatically, by 419% and 244% respectively (Sloan *et al*, 1986, p. 31). The cost for a coronary bypass in 1987 was "in excess of $25,000 per procedure" at Medicare rates (Evans 1991, p. 64). The total cost of uncomplicated hip arthroplasties escalated from $690 million in 1979 to almost $4 billion in 1985 (Evans 1991, p. 65). A number of other surgical procedures have also showed significant increases: for example, the number of heart transplants, which cost anywhere from $200,00 to $400,000 each depending on the severity of complications (Menzel 1990, p. 170), increased from

62 in 1981 to 1,647 in 1988 (Evans 1991, p. 57). Cataract surgery was up 207% and surgery for morbid obesity was up 132% (Sloan *et al*, 1986, pp. 31-32). In addition, kidney transplants, which now number 9000 annually (Menzel 1990, p. 169), would also rise were it not for the shortage of donors. Liver transplants, which cost at least $150,000 and which numbered 200 in 1984, increased to 900 by 1986 (Menzel 1990, p. 169), and there are estimates that "40,000 people are plausible candidates" (Menzel 1990, p. 170).

Furthermore, cardiac transplants are being carried out on older people. In the United States, between 1973 and 1983, there were only 13 people over the age of 55 who had a cardiac transplant. By 1986 that number had increased to 249 (Evans 1991, p. 58). The annual cost of kidney dialysis in the United States rose from $229 million in 1974 to $1.3 billion in 1980 and to over $3 billion in 1990 (Evans 1991, p. 49). Like cardiac transplants, "persons aged 65 and older are the fastest-growing age group in the dialysis population, increasing at an annual rate of over 15 percent" (Evans 1991, p. 49).

Furthermore, the survival rate of each of these high-tech transplants and procedures is steadily improving, especially since the introduction of cyclosporine in the 1980s. Before 1980 cardiac transplants had, on average, a one-year survival rate of only 64% and a five-year survival rate of 39%. With the advent of cyclosporine one-year and five-year survival rates for cardiac transplants increased, respectively, to 87% and 53% (Evans 1991, p. 57).

Kidney transplants, when successful, are now more cost effective than dialysis. The average cost of a kidney transplant is $41,045, with annual follow-up costs ranging from $6,000 to $11,000. Dialysis, on the other hand, costs $25,000 per year (Evans 1991, p. 53). Thus over a ten-year period the cost of a transplant, including the maximum estimated follow-up costs, would be $151,045 as compared to the $250,000 of renal dialysis. Moreover, as the technology for developing artificial organs improves, the shortage of organs will no longer be a problem and there will be an increased demand for what medicine, in conjunction with the new technology, can offer.

In addition, there is the problem of people who not only contribute to their own morbidity and mortality through various high risk activities but also contribute to increased health care expenditures for the rest of the population. Consider, for example, smoking. A recent study has concluded that "$187 billion, 18% of medical expenditures, can be taken as the premium currently being paid every five years to provide medical care for the excess disease suffered by smokers" (Hodgson 1992, p. 111). That amount is $54.10 billion greater than the $132.9 billion spent on health care in the United States in 1975. Of course, we have all heard of the dangers of smoking, but, nonetheless, people continue to smoke, and continue to start to smoke,[61] despite evidence that it is directly responsible for 21% of the deaths from heart disease, or 115,00 deaths per year (Manson *et al*, 1992, p. 1406). In this latter study Manson and colleagues estimated the reduction in risk for myocardial infarctions that could be achieved by altering one's lifestyle. They found that by simply quitting smoking, people could reduce the risk of myocardial infarction anywhere from 50 to 70% (Manson *et al*, 1992, p. 1407); by maintaining an active lifestyle or an ideal body weight, between 35 to 55% (Manson *et al*, 1992, p. 1410 and p. 1411); reducing alcohol intake to mild-to-moderate consumption, between 25 to 45%; and for women, postmenopausal estrogen therapy could reduce their risk by 44% (Manson *et al*, 1992, p. 1412). In addition to these measures, there are other personal behaviors that consistently have been found to promote health: an adequate amount of sleep, eating breakfast, not eating between meals, and getting and staying married.

Daniels notes that there is "nothing in [his] view [that] makes health protection so overriding a concern that we may deny individuals the autonomy to take risks that endanger life, liver, and lungs" (Daniels 1985, p. 153). Therefore, while he may not endorse high risk activity, he permits it, as he should, but the people who engage in such activities are not made to pay the cost of their engaging in these behaviors. The problem is not simply that people engage in high risk activities, thereby increasing the costs all must pay and thus free-ride on their more health conscious neighbors, although this is important. But rather the problem is that there is no means available to Daniels' theory that could limit the number of people engaging in such high risk activities, and therefore this can only add to the severity of the supply problem. In addition to excessive consumption of alcohol and smoking, there are numerous other high risk activities that people can and do engage in; some may be innocent activities, while others may not. These other activities can range from drug abuse and unprotected sexual intercourse to playing amateur and/or professional sports, from being employed in certain occupations -- such as mining or handling dangerous materials -- to failing to exercise due care and attention when driving.

In addition to the morbidity and the supply problem, Daniels' fair equality of opportunity argument fails to include a principled means to either circumvent or mitigate the problem of ensuring that the cost of medical and/or diagnostic treatments does not outweigh the benefits. Daniels maintains that prevention of disease is as important, if not more important, than treatment. Recall that on Daniels' four-tier health care delivery system preventive health care is the first tier. Its function is to minimize departures from the ideal of species-typical normal functioning, but the important question is, at what cost? Consider the estimated cost for one preventive measure, screening for colorectal cancer.

In 1974 the American Cancer Society advanced the idea that six guaiac tests -- an inexpensive test for detecting small amounts of blood in a person's stool -- be used to screen for colorectal cancer. After careful analysis, based on the assumption that the initial test cost $4.00 and that the cost of each additional test cost $1.00 and taking into account the fact that each subsequent test produced fewer results in terms of the number of cases of cancer detected, it was determined that the marginal cost per case of detected cancer increased exponentially. For one test to detect just one case of colorectal cancer would cost $1175; it would cost $5492 for two tests to detect another case; $49,150 for three tests to detect a third case; $469,534 for four tests to detect a fourth case; $4.7 million for five tests to detect a fifth case; and just over $47 million for the full six test screen to detect but one case, albeit the sixth case (Neuhauser and Lewicki, 1975, p. 227).[62] Note that these dollar values reflect not the cost of treating the cancer once it has been detected but rather only the cost of detecting it. One should note that the main reason for the escalating costs is that for each test performed, fewer and fewer cases of this type of cancer would be detected; that is, while the cost per test is very small, the cost for detecting each case of colorectal cancer is not.

Presumably part of what it means to have access to one's normal opportunity range is not to die prematurely from diseases which can be detected. But, as the above example shows, the cost of simply detecting but one case of a disease which could result in premature death, never mind the cost of treating the disease once it has been detected, is prohibitively expensive. If a society is to ensure fair equality of opportunity by providing for all of its citizens to have access to their normal opportunity range, then it must engage in some preventive health care. Indeed, on Daniels' account, preventive health care is the first tier of his four-tier system of health care delivery, and while he may claim that "it is preferable to prevent than to have to cure, and to cure than to have to compensate for lost functioning" (Daniels 1985, p. 48), he also says that both the institutions and services of at least three of the four tiers "are needed if fair equality of opportunity is to be guaranteed" (Daniels 1985, p. 48). One might also note that to the extent that preventive, as well as curative, measures are efficacious, we would face a further drain on the remainder of a society's resources, for longer lives would surely involve more consumption but not, unfortunately, more productivity.

The people who suffer the most in terms of deviations from the norm of species-typical normal functioning are those that are the most sick and/or injured. Therefore it will be those people whose normal opportunity range will be most adversely affected. And if, as Daniels claims, the "moral function of the health care system must be" (Daniels 1985, p. 41) to help guarantee fair equality of opportunity, then it is those people who will have the greatest claim on our health care system. If their claims cannot be constrained by some mechanism within his theory, then they will consume the vast majority of health care, leaving little or none for the remainder of the population who could benefit.

Rawls constrained the scope of his fair equality of opportunity principle in two distinct ways, neither of which is open to Daniels. The first way Rawls constrained the scope of his fair equality of opportunity principle was by the lexical ordering of the principles of justice. This requires that we satisfy all the requirements of the first principle prior to satisfying the requirements of the next principle. The difference principle was the second way Rawls constrained the scope of his fair equality of opportunity principle. The difference principle instructs us to equalize opportunity up to that point at which the least advantaged are made as well off as possible.

Neither of these two Rawlsian alternatives are available to

Daniels, and for three reasons. First, Daniels has eschewed not only any appeal to the other Rawlsian principles of justice, but also any appeals to Rawls' general theory of justice as fairness. Daniels cannot appeal to the lexical ordering of the principles of justice for his account of justice in health care only appeals to the principle of fair equality of opportunity and thus there is no other principle that could be lexically prior to the principle of fair equality of opportunity. In addition, Daniels claims that his argument does not "depend on the acceptability of any particular theory of justice," (Daniels 1985, pp. 41) let alone Rawls'.Hence Daniels takes it to be the case that his argument will stand or fall on its own merits.

It is of course possible that Daniels holds that there is another principle, or principles, of justice to which he might appeal. For the sake of argument, let us assume there is some other principle. If he did appeal to some other principle, for example the liberty principle, then he would face two problems. The first problem Daniels would face would be deciding on how the principles ought to be ordered if they could not be satisfied simultaneously. Then, regardless of the order chosen, one principle would have priority over the other. If the liberty principle had priority over the fair equality of opportunity principle, then (when both principles could not be satisfied) the liberty principle would have priority and health care would lose its status and a "special social good" (Daniels 1985, p. 56). If the fair equality of opportunity principle had priority over the liberty principle, then (again when both principles could not be satisfied), while health care would retain its status as a "special social good," we would find our liberty restricted for reasons other than that we were harming others.[63] And while Daniels could accept restricting people's liberty in order to prevent them from harming others, he would not accept restricting people's liberty in order to enlarge their opportunity range. For, as we noted earlier, there is nothing in Daniels' view that "makes health protection so overriding a concern that we may deny individuals the autonomy to take risks that endanger life, liver, and lungs" (Daniels 1985, p. 153).

Daniels does attempt to provide constraints for the scope of his broader conception of fair equality of opportunity in two ways. He first argues that the principle of fair equality of opportunity defines "from the perspective of justice, what the moral function of the health care system must be -- to help guarantee fair equality of opportunity" (Daniels 1985, p. 41). He then argues "health-care institutions have the limited function of maintaining normal species functioning: they eliminate individual differences due only to disease or disability" (Daniels 1985, p. 53). Finally, he argues that he is concerned, not with the effective opportunity range -- that is, "the share of the normal range determined by an individual's actual choices about what life plans to pursue and talents and skills to develop" (Daniels 1985, p. 47), but rather what he calls the normal opportunity range; that is, "the array of life plans reasonable persons in [the society] are likely to construct for themselves" (Daniels 1985, p. 33), "not the ones he actually does" (Daniels 1985, p. 47).

Daniels' first response does little in the way of resolving the morbidity problem, and for at least two reasons. The first reason is that it is not the case that the fair equality of opportunity principle defines what the moral function of the health care system must be. Most people, we would think, would say that the moral function of the health care system "from the perspective of justice" is to aid the sick, the injured, and the dying, not to mention research and development, education, and gate keeping functions (Friedson 1986, chap. 4). In addition, our health care system takes on these roles completely independently of whether or not such activity affects our opportunity range.[64] The second reason Daniels' response does little in the way of solving the morbidity problem is that if it were true that the moral function of a health care system is to protect equality of opportunity, then it must first protect the opportunities of those who need it most; that is, those who are so sick and/or injured that they can benefit in terms of improving and/or protecting their normal opportunity range. But those who are so sick and/or injured, are also the most expensive to care for.

Daniels attempts to constrain the scope of his fair equality of opportunity argument, such that he might avoid the restricted version of the morbidity problem, in a second way. He argues that his fair equality of opportunity account of justice in health care is concerned not with the effective opportunity range, but rather only the normal opportunity range. The problem with this approach is similar to the problem of the first approach. While it may preclude specific individuals from claiming a moral right to a specific medical treatment or procedure in order to pursue a specific life plan (for example, cosmetic surgery so that one can be a model or a news anchor), it does not exempt Daniels' fair equality of opportunity argument from addressing the true nature of the restricted version of the morbidity problem. That is, there are some people, say 9% of the population, who are sick and/or injured but who can still benefit in terms of improving and/or protecting their normal (as opposed to their effective) opportunity range, who have, not only a moral claim on the health care resources of a society committed to guaranteeing fair equality of opportunity, but a weightier moral claim than their less opportunity-restricted fellows. Moreover, as we demonstrated above, this proportion of the population consumes the vast majority of health care resources.

Daniels notes that his account of the four-tiered health care delivery is not meant to imply "that each layer corresponds to a particular principle of justice, or that the layers are ranked in moral priority" (Daniels 1985, p. 48). However, given that we have only a limited amount of resources that can be devoted to all social programs in the name of fair equality of opportunity, we first need to ensure that the amount ultimately devoted to health care does not detract from society's other efforts to protect and/or achieve fair equality of opportunity. This assumes, of course, that health care does not take priority over all efforts to protect and/or achieve fair equality of opportunity, an issue on which Daniels is silent. Notwithstanding this latter problem, let us assume that there is an amount that is solely devoted to health care and that this allocated amount was decided upon in conjunction with the other social efforts that attempt to protect and/or achieve fair equality of opportunity.

On Daniels' account society is supposed to devise health care institutions within the constraints of this allocated amount. The problem which now remains is that we need some principle for ranking how these health care dollars ought to be spent so that we achieve maximum results. One might think that we could look at any preventive, curative, or maintenance measure and ascertain the marginal benefits of each of the proposed alternatives. However, without some account of who is actually the worse off in terms of restrictions of their opportunity range, assuming that the worst off have priority, society could not decide which of any of the proposed alternatives would provide the most in terms of marginal benefits. For example, who is to say that persons needing cardiac transplants are worse off than people needing a different organ, when, if neither gets the organ, death results. Or, who is worse off, people who have contracted the AIDS virus and will die within a few years, or people who have Huntington's Chorea, a disease that typically does not manifest itself until (approximately) mid-life? Examples such as these could be multiplied but two will suffice, for they demonstrate the need for some principle that can be appealed to in order to answer such questions, a principle which is lacking in Daniels' argument.

The problem of determining who is worse off in terms of restrictions on their opportunity range, as well as the problem of containing health care expenditures so as to avoid the bottomless pit, is compounded by the expansiveness of what constitutes health care needs in Daniels' theory. Recall that he included, among other things, life-style features such as exercise and rest, and nutrition and shelter. The problem is further compounded without some account of personal responsibility. For example, does an adult crack addict have a weightier claim to health care resources than a crack-addicted baby, given that the latter had no say in contracting the condition and the former did? These deficiencies, as well as Daniels' failure to provide a device within his theory to resolve any one of the three aspects of the bottomless pit problem, raise serious doubts as to the acceptability of Daniels' theory of justice in health care.

However, assuming he could find the resources within his theory to mitigate these deficiencies, his argument would still suffer from the difficulty of, paradoxically, narrowing ranges of opportunity. Presumably, on Daniels' account, the money for funding health care would be raised through taxation. Either the money raised through taxation would be sufficient to meet annual health care expenditures or it would not. If the money raised through taxation was sufficient to meet annual health care expenditures, then people would have less money to spend on their other non-health care preferences. This assumes, of course, that people have limited resources such that they cannot satisfy all their preferences. If people have less money to spend on their other non-health care related preferences, because of the amount they are taxed to fund Daniels' theory of justice in health care, then they will be unable to satisfy the preferences they would have satisfied if they had not been taxed the amount necessary to fund annual health care expenditures. Furthermore, if one's opportunity range is related to these non-health care preferences, then, to the extent that one cannot satisfy one's preferences, one's opportunity range has been restricted. If the money raised through taxation was insufficient to meet the annual health care budget, then, the remaining funds would, presumably, be raised through deficit financing; that is, raising the national debt to provide for the amount necessary to meet the annual health care budget. If this were the case, then while the opportunity range of the present generation might not be narrowed, the opportunity range of some future generation or generations would be narrowed. The opportunity range of some future generation or generations would be narrowed on the assumption that deficit financing cannot be continued indefinitely. Thus, on either account, we would end up with a narrowing of opportunity ranges, either the range of the present generation or the range of some future generation or generations.

Daniels defines the concept of a normal opportunity range as "the array of life plans reasonable persons in [the society] are likely to construct for themselves" (Daniels 1985, p. 33). Our preceding argument rests on this same definition. The life plans reasonable persons in a society are likely to construct for themselves are just those plans that people make with respect to educating themselves, choosing a career, having a family, providing for their children's education, and providing for their retirement. If the amount that people are taxed in order to fund annual health care expenditures is greater than the amount that they would have voluntarily spent on health care, then they will have less money to spend on these other areas. For example, if the amount a person was taxed in order to fund annual health care expenditures was greater than the amount he would have been willing to pay for health care insurance, then that person might be unable to afford to attend a better university and/or to send his children to a private rather than a public school. Consequently, his range of opportunity would be less than it would be in the absence of the tax necessary to fund annual health care expenditures.

The final problem we will address with respect to Daniels' fair equality of opportunity argument for justice in health care, and which is directly related to the fundamental problem with Daniels' approach sketched above, is tied to his reliance on Boorse's biomedical model of disease (Boorse 1981). Our concern here is not give a detailed criticism of the Daniels-cum-Boorse biomedical model of disease, of how such an account presupposes that one must analyze disease in terms of dysfunctions, as opposed to either "action failures" (Fulford 1989, pp. 109-140) or the failure of Boorse's account to include "the role of inclusive fitness in [his] evolutionary accounts of 'biological design'" (Engelhardt 1986, pp. 168). Rather our concern is merely to show that some people value what health care has to offer for reasons which are, at least sometimes, completely independent of the question of disease. Some conditions for which people seek out medical treatment are not diseases, yet people value the services provided by the medical practitioner at least as much as they would value some of the services of a practitioner who provided disease related services to them. For example, even though fertility is normal in terms of species typical functioning, sterility is not. However, if one did not value paternity, then one would have a good reason for valuing the services of the doctor who provided a vasectomy.[65] There are numerous other examples that could also be cited: the person seeking a sex change operation values both the surgery and the requisite supply of drugs to effect the change and neither is abnormal in terms of species typical functioning; pregnancy, aging, adolescent puberty changes, drug and alcohol problems, and abortions are all not diseases on Daniels' model, and yet people value the medical services which responds to their particular wants with respect to these conditions.

Daniels' account of the biomedical model of disease is unable to account for these and many more conditions that are valued, or disvalued as the case may be, but are not diseases. What is important for these people may have little or nothing to do with whether their particular concern is a disease or not. What is important for these people is that they have certain wants, values, plans and, to use Lomasky's term, projects (Lomasky 1987, chap. 2). They have a conception of what constitutes the good life for them and they want to have access to the means which will allow them to achieve it. Of course, Daniels' fair equality of opportunity argument does not rule out, although it does restrict, the possibility that people could pay their own way with respect to achieving any of the particular non-disease but medically related values. But that is not the important point. The important point with respect to Daniels' biomedical model of disease is that it fails to account for a great deal of what people actually and reasonably want and/or desire when they seek medical attention.

We conclude this chapter by identifying some of the more important lessons we have learned from Daniels attempt to do justice in health care. We have learned about the bottomless pit problem and the three aspects which make it especially troubling: the morbidity problem, the supply problem, and the cost/benefit problem. In addition, we have identified some of the empirical evidence that makes these problems real, rather than just theoretical problems. Furthermore, in order to resolve these problems, we have learned that a theory of justice in health care needs to provide some mechanism or device within the theory for constraining the consumption of health care, lest health care consumes all of our resources.

Health maintenance is, at least in part, a personal responsibility. To the extent that people are allowed the liberty to engage in unhealthy behaviors, they increase the costs the rest of society must bear. Daniels' theory, to its credit, does not deny that people may engage in risky and/or unhealthy behavior. However, his theory lacks any mechanism or device for relegating these unnecessary costs to the parties responsible. Without such a mechanism, the cost of engaging in these behaviors is displaced among all members of society, which results in free-riding by some at the expense of others.

Finally, health care is important, as Daniels has argued. However, the importance of health care lies not just in the physician's ability to correct for deviations from species-typical functioning. More significantly, health care is important because it is a means to the achievement of goals or projects we may have, one of which is undoubtably good health itself. However, while health care is important, so are many other things, and especially to those with limited resources. Daniels, in attempting to tie health care to opportunity, neglected to consider the opportunity costs of doing so. Once we account for these opportunity costs it is clear that a theory that seeks to guarantee fair equality of opportunity by providing health care can do so only at the completely unacceptable price of, paradoxically, restricting one's opportunity range.

With these lessons in mind, we turn to Allen Buchanan's contribution. Because Buchanan's argument is different in form, content, and conclusions, some of the problems his argument will face will be different than the one's identified in this chapter.

Chapter IV

Enforced Beneficence and the Decent Minimum Project

In the previous chapter we examined Norman Daniels' fair equality of opportunity argument for justice in health care, and we found the argument lacking in several respects. In particular we found that his theory did not contain any mechanism which was sufficient to constrain the consumption of health care and thus avoid any one of the three aspects of the theory-dependent version of the bottomless pit problem. Penultimately, we also argued that, pace Daniels, attempting to use health care to guarantee fair equality of opportunity need not result in an increase in the scope of one's opportunity range, but rather, paradoxically, could result in a decrease in the scope of one's opportunity range. We concluded our criticism of Daniels' fair equality of opportunity argument by arguing that while his theory may indeed take care of people's medical needs, it did not take care of people's medical wants and/or desires.

We now turn our attention to the promissory note we made near the beginning of the last chapter. We suggested earlier that Daniels' admitted concession, that his theory could not cover everyone and in particular those who could not benefit in terms of their opportunity range, might gain some needed support from Buchanan's enforced beneficence arguments. Buchanan, with these arguments, attempts to show that "there is a sound justification for an enforced principle guaranteeing a decent minimum of health care to everyone" (Buchanan 1984, p. 66). If he is successful, then not only would Buchanan provide additional support for Daniels' argument, assuming Daniels' argument could be modified to overcome our earlier objections, Buchanan will have made an important contribution to the issue of justice in health care in his own right. Furthermore, if Buchanan's arguments are successful, he will have demonstrated that there is a positive right to health care while avoiding the problems that Daniels' argument faced.

For example, rather than seeking to defend a universal right to health care in the traditional sense, Buchanan attempts to find a number of arguments which, he suggests, will "do the work of an alleged universal right to a decent minimum of health care" (Buchanan 1984, p. 66). Second, given that Buchanan is only arguing for "an enforced principle guaranteeing a decent minimum of health care to everyone" (Buchanan 1984, p. 66), rather than a universal right to health care *per se*, he should be able to avoid the three aspects of the bottomless pit problem to which Daniels' argument succumbed. Finally, assuming that his arguments are sound and that the concept of a decent minimum can be satisfactorily defined, his contribution to our present concern is important for he will have identified an important new strategy for resolving certain kinds of public policy issues.

Buchanan begins his argument by distinguishing between a universal rights-claim and a special rights-claim. The former is generally understood to mean that all persons have the right in question, whereas the latter is understood to mean that the right in question is restricted to "certain individuals or groups" (Buchanan 1984, p. 67). Buchanan's purpose for drawing this distinction is that he wants to argue that

> the combined weight of arguments from special (as opposed to universal) rights to health care, harm prevention, prudential arguments of the sort used to justify public health measures, and two arguments that show that effective charity shares features of public goods (in the technical sense) is sufficient to do the work of an alleged universal right to a decent minimum of health care (Buchanan 1984, p. 67).

Although Buchanan alludes to several types of arguments that could be made to support a right to a decent minimum of health care, he actually presents only two arguments, his two enforced beneficence arguments. Nor does he offer any actual arguments in place of these alluded-to arguments in an earlier version of this same paper (Buchanan 1983).

In the place of particular arguments for what he terms "arguments from special rights" (Buchanan 1984, p. 66) we have only an allusion to "three types of arguments that can be given for special rights to health care" (Buchanan 1984, p. 67), all of which are compensatory justice arguments: an argument for rectifying past and/or present injustices, an argument requiring compensation from those who unjustly expose innocent people to various health risks, and an argument to the effect that those who were wounded in military service should be entitled to some health care services as a means of compensating them for their injuries.

In the place of particular arguments for what he terms "arguments from the prevention of harms" he merely suggests that a harm prevention principle could go some distance in supporting a social policy of providing "basic health care services [which] should not vary greatly across different racial, ethnic, or geographic groups within the country" (Buchanan 1984, p. 68). Finally, with respect to what he terms "prudential arguments," he again merely suggests that "the availability of certain basic forms of health care make for a more productive labor force or improve the fitness of the citizenry for national defense" (Buchanan 1984, p. 68).

The only substantive arguments Buchanan makes in favor of a right to a decent minimum of health care are his two enforced beneficence arguments. As Buchanan suggested in the above quoted passage, the merit of his pluralistic approach was purported to be that the combined weight of all of these types of arguments would do the work of an alleged universal right to a decent minimum of health care. However, this could only be the case if the latter two arguments for enforced beneficence were sound and if the alluded-to arguments could carry the moral and/or legal weight which he implies can be found in them. Since Buchanan does not offer any particular arguments in support of his claim that the sorts of arguments he alludes to would do the work of an alleged universal right to a decent minimum of health care, we shall not consider them here. Instead, we shall focus our attention on Buchanan's two enforced beneficence arguments.

Buchanan premises his two enforced beneficence arguments on the assumption that "there is a basic moral obligation of charity or beneficence to those in need" (Buchanan 1984, p. 69).

He then goes on to argue, in the first argument, that even if people recognize and are "motivationally capable of acting" (Buchanan 1984, p. 70) so as to fulfil their moral obligation to provide for those in need, they might not do so. The reason for their possible failure to contribute, he argues, is not *akrasia* (or weakness of will) but rather their rationality.

Suppose, Buchanan assumes, that we recognize that a collective effort to establish a decent minimum of health care for all is "a more important form of beneficence than the various charitable acts A, B, and C" (Buchanan 1984, p. 70).[66] If we are rational, Buchanan argues, we will each reason as follows:

> either enough others will contribute to the decent minimum project to achieve this goal, even if I do not contribute to it; or not enough others will contribute to achieve a decent minimum, even if I do contribute. In either case, my contribution will be wasted" (Buchanan 1984, p. 70).

One's contribution would be wasted for the reason that, given "the virtually negligible size of my own contribution" (Buchanan 1984, p. 70), one's own contribution will neither make nor break the project. Hence, each individual concludes that since his own contribution would be wasted, he could better fulfill his obligation of charity if he performed some individual act of charity, such as giving his particular contribution to some particular needy person. Thus, the argument goes, even though all recognize that a joint effort to establish the decent minimum project is the best way to fulfill one's charitable duty, given the rationality of each individual, each will fail to contribute and the decent minimum project will not be realized. The way to resolve this problem, Buchanan argues, is to force every one to contribute. By doing so we would ensure that, despite our rationality, we would achieve the goal we all admit that we want to accomplish.

This argument is a form of the standard public goods argument. A public good (in the technical sense that Buchanan referred to earlier) has two key properties, indivisibility and non-excludability. That is, if a good is indivisible, then, if it is made available to one person, it is equally available to all. The non-excludability property of a public good means that it is not feasible or efficient to exclude people (i.e., those who do not pay) from consuming the good.[67] In the standard public goods argument, some argue that collective action is necessary to achieve the good in question. If we assume that people are individually rational, then the desired public good might not be produced for it might not be individually rational for each person to contribute to its production. It might not be individually rational for each person to contribute to the production of a public good for at least two reasons. The first reason is that people may lack the assurance that others will contribute and thus realize the decent minimum project. The second reason it might not be individually rational for each person to contribute is that if the good in question is nonexclusive -- that is, no one can be prevented from consuming it -- then it is possible that each person will be able to consume the good in question, assuming it is produced, without bearing any of the costs in producing it. In other words, he will be able to free-ride. We shall refer to these two possible reasons for not contributing as, respectively, the assurance problem and the free rider problem (Schmidtz 1991, p. 56).

In Buchanan's version of the public goods argument, each individual fails to contribute because he lacks assurance others will also contribute. Thus, while each individual might be concerned to maximize the amount of good he could achieve with his limited beneficence budget, unless each individual has assurance that others will also contribute, it would not be rational for a particular individual to contribute to the decent minimum project. That is, given that a particular individual's contribution to the decent minimum project will be wasted, whether he contributes or not, he reasons that the rational and the most beneficent thing to do is not contribute to the joint effort but rather to undertake an individual charitable act. But if all reasoned this way, the decent minimum project, which by assumption is a more important form of beneficence than individual charitable acts, will not be realized. Buchanan's solution to the assurance problem is simple, force all to contribute to the decent minimum project.

Buchanan's second argument is closely related to the first argument, albeit with significant differences. Once again he assumes that securing a decent minimum is more important than particular individual acts of charity. He also assumes that people are willing to contribute to the decent minimum project but only if they have assurance that enough others will also contribute. Without such assurance, he argues, it would not be rational to contribute to the decent minimum project, for if there is no such assurance one's contribution would be wasted. Therefore, he concludes, the rational thing to do would be to expend one's beneficence budget by performing some other particular act of charity. But if everyone spent their budget on individual acts of charity the end result would not be as good as it would be if all contributed to the decent minimum project. Finally, he concludes, in order to resolve the problem of individual contributions being wasted, we should all be forced to contribute.

While these two arguments may seem to be powerful arguments, they do not accomplish what Buchanan thinks they do; that is, they do not provide a sound justification for an enforcement mechanism to ensure charitable contributions. Buchanan has not argued that actual people would not or do not make actual charitable contributions, rather his theoretical point is that rational people, where rationality is defined in terms of maximizing one's expected utility, would not make such contributions. Thus if we merely focused on the empirical evidence to the contrary, we would fail to give Buchanan's more substantial philosophical point its due. Moreover, not only did we suggest that Buchanan's argument might be used to supplement the admitted weakness in Daniels' fair equality of opportunity argument, his approach, if successful, will provide an important new view on how we might resolve certain kinds of public policy issues.

Let us suppose, for the sake of argument, that Buchanan's first enforced beneficence argument is valid. If it is valid then, as Buchanan argued, we need an enforcement mechanism, presumably the state, to ensure everyone contributes. But if, as Buchanan argued, an individual's contribution would be wasted in the event that he voluntarily contributed to the decent minimum project, then we need some reason for thinking that an individual's contribution would not be wasted if it was forcibly taken from him by the state. At first glance, Buchanan seems to offer no reason for thinking that would not be the case. The assumption made by Buchanan, with respect to a person's voluntary contribution being wasted even if enough others also voluntarily contributed to the decent minimum project, was that "granted the scale of the investment required and the virtually negligible size of my own contribution, I can disregard the minute possibility that my contribution might make the difference between [the] success [or] failure" (Buchanan 1984, p. 70) of the decent minimum project. But if an individual's contribution will not make the difference between the success or failure of the decent minimum project when it comes to voluntarily contributing to the decent minimum project, will it make the difference between the success or failure of the decent minimum project when it comes to state-enforced individual contributions? On Buchanan's account, yes.

The government, by coercing people to contribute to the decent minimum project, resolves the two assurance problems that concern Buchanan. Enforced contributions ensures that enough people will contribute to the decent minimum project and it ensures that the amount of contributions is sufficient to meet the demands of the decent minimum project, whatever they might amount to. Thus, on the one hand, Buchanan's argument, if successful, resolves two substantive problems of strategic rationality, the problem of ensuring that enough people will contribute and the problem of ensuring that the amount of contributions are sufficient to meet the demands of the decent minimum project. On the other hand, however, even if Buchanan's argument is successful, we have little or no reason for thinking that one universal project of providing health care will fare any better than the disaggregated system now in place in the United States, an issue we shall return to shortly.

Buchanan's two arguments are meant to demonstrate that it would not be rational for people to contribute voluntarily to the decent minimum project. What his argument has not shown, and what it must show if his overall project is to go through, is that a coercive mechanism for ensuring contributions to the decent minimum project is the only available means for resolving both problems identified above. In addition, Buchanan must also show that political solutions, such as enforced contributions, are less costly than either social solutions or moral solutions.

David Schmidtz has argued for a social solution to the assurance problem. Schmidtz's solution is what he calls an "assurance contract," or a "contractual agreement to contribute to a public goods project" (Schmidtz 1991, p. 66). The essential feature of Schmidtz's assurance contract is that the contractual agreement "need only specify, for each particular party, what consideration is expected from the parties involved as a group" (Schmidtz 1991, p. 66; italics in the original). Thus, suppose we were concerned to realize the decent minimum project. If everyone who was expected to contribute had the assurance that all who were expected to contribute would contribute and the assurance that the amount collected would be sufficient for the decent minimum project to be realized, then no one's contribution would be wasted and the decent minimum project would be realized. Buchanan's political solution, enforced contributions, provides both these assurances and therefore under his account the decent minimum project could be realized. But suppose further, as Schmidtz does, that rather than forcing people to contribute, we offer them a "money-back guarantee" (Schmidtz 1991, p. 66). That is, suppose we guarantee to all who would be expected to contribute to the decent minimum project that if either everyone who was expected to contribute did not contribute, and/or that if the amount collected was insufficient to meet the demands of the decent minimum project, then all monies would be returned. With these assurances, people would, Schmidtz argues, voluntarily contribute to the production of public goods.

That people would voluntarily contribute to the production of public goods, given the existence of assurance contracts, is important for it demonstrates that there are alternatives to Buchanan's political solution to the assurance problem. Therefore, Buchanan's conclusion, that people ought to be forced to contribute to the decent minimum project, does not follow from his premises; that is, his argument is invalid. The most that Buchanan could conclude from his premises is that some mechanism is needed to resolve the assurance problem. In order to conclude that this mechanism must be an enforced mechanism, Buchanan must show either that political solutions are less costly than non-political solutions or that there are no non-political solutions. We have identified a non-political solution, Schmidtz's social solution of assurance contracts, that is a viable alternative to Buchanan's political solution to the assurance problem. However, we have not demonstrated that Schmidtz's social solution is less costly than Buchanan's political solution and we will not attempt such a demonstration, for showing that Buchanan's conclusion is not the only conclusion that can be reached is sufficient for undermining his argument. We now want to turn our attention to other aspects of Buchanan's argument which are equally troubling.

The concept of a decent minimum of health care has been conspicuously avoided up until now, for we wanted to demonstrate that Buchanan's argument failed independently of the decent minimum concept. It is unclear from the text what Buchanan means by a decent minimum. All he says is that

> those who favor the non-rights-based approach can argue that the difficulty encountered by rights-based approaches in specifying the content of an alleged right to a decent minimum provides indirect support for the position that there is no right to a decent minimum but only an enforceable duty of beneficence or charity to contribute to the attainment of a decent minimum. In other words, the advocate of the enforced beneficence approach can warmly welcome the lack of a principled specification as a vindication of his view rather than accept it begrudgingly as an embarrassing theoretical lacuna. The idea would be that we must frankly acknowledge that the character and scope of the list of services included in the decent minimum is a matter of collective choice. All that is necessary is that there be some fair procedure for reaching a social decision on which set of services to provide (Buchanan 1984, pp. 77-78).

Such a response is inadequate for a number of reasons. The most important reason is that, even if his beneficence arguments demonstrated that there was a duty of enforced beneficence, which they could not, Buchanan would still need to show that the duty of enforced beneficence entailed providing the amount that is necessary for a decent minimum. For, even if we grant that we have a duty of beneficence, enforced or otherwise, it does not follow from this, without further substantive argument, that we must therefore contribute the amount necessary for providing a decent minimum of health care. It may be the case that the amount our duty of beneficence requires is substantially less than what would constitute a decent minimum, unless, of course, by decent Buchanan means something other than what we took it to mean.

Thus far we have taken the phrase 'decent minimum of health care' to mean roughly an adequate amount of health care. However, the concept "decent" has normative content as well. It can mean, for example, conformity with a standard of conduct or propriety. On this account to say that people were entitled to a decent minimum of health care would mean little more than to say that they were entitled to only what we choose to give them. If this is what Buchanan meant by a decent minimum of health care, then it may not be sufficient to meet people's basic health care needs.

Moreover, even if we concede that there is a duty of beneficence, Buchanan's argument, because it !acks any sort of connection between beneficence and health care, tells us nothing
specifically about health care, yet his argument rests on there
being such a connection. Without a conceptual connection between beneficence and health care, the notion of a decent minimum of health care is opaque and therefore can play no major
role in Buchanan's argument. Health care is but one form of aid.
There are many others, alms to the poor, food to the hungry,
shelter for the homeless, to mention just a few. And, even if one
could establish that our duty of beneficence required the provision of health care services, as opposed to these other forms of
aid, it still would not follow that the amount required was
sufficient to meet the demands of a decent minimum, understood
in the former sense.

One would have thought that the content of a decent minimum would be somehow tied to what people actually need rather
than what we collectively choose to give them. For it may be the
case that what we collectively choose to give people may not be
what they need. If what we collectively choose to give people is
not what they need, then how can it be said that we are providing
them with a decent minimum?

Buchanan's argument rests on there being a connection between three concepts, beneficence, decency, and health care, and
while there might be such a connection, Buchanan has not
demonstrated it. Therefore, even if Buchanan's enforced beneficence arguments were successful, they would have told us
nothing specific about rights to health care, let alone a positive
right to a decent minimum of health care. Moreover, as some
empirical evidence seems to show, not only is it the case that a
universal project of ensuring health care for all may not be better
than the disagregated system now in place in the United States,
but also there may be more important determining factors of
good health than the contributions made by the medical establishment. If further research supports this general observation,
then we will need some further arguments from Buchanan as to
why our basic moral duty of beneficence did not pertain to these
alternative factors rather than health care *per se.*

The most common arguments being advanced today for a
universal approach to providing health care are made by comparing the U.S.'s health care delivery system with that of other

countries, and most specifically Canada. On the positive side, as we noted in our comparative analysis of the Canadian and American health care delivery systems, we found, among other things, that per capita health care expenditures were lower in Canada than in the U.S, that the percentage of GNP spent on health care in Canada was less than that of the United States, that Canadians were generally more pleased with their system of health care than Americans were, and that everyone was insured for medical care, while in the United States over 30 million are uninsured. On the negative side, we found, again among other things, that Canada has substantially fewer pieces of high-tech medical equipment per capita than the U.S., substantially fewer facilities for performing the latest high-tech medical procedures, and that the U.S. provides an outlet for Canadians when they cannot breach the limits imposed on the delivery of some health care services by their universal system of health care delivery.

In addition, in the previous chapter we argued that, pace Daniels, not only was it not the case that tying health care to a fair equality of opportunity principle necessarily increased one's opportunity range, but that such a move could decrease one's opportunity range. One's opportunity range could be decreased, we argued, because tying health care to the fair equality of opportunity principle might give people more health care insurance than what they might rationally want to purchase. This, we argued, resulted in precluding some individuals from trading off their future health care consumption against some of their more pressing present preferences and/or forgoing some of those preferences due to a lack of funds. Thus if the decent minimum project were implemented, then Americans, like their Canadian counterparts, would also suffer from this same problem; American's current opportunity of trading off future health care consumption against other more pressing present preferences would be eliminated.

In addition to these reasons, as noted in a JAMA editorial, there is evidence to suggest that "there seems to be little relationship between the percentage of gross national product spent on medical and health care and the extent of improvements in expected life span" (Lundberg 1992, p. 2522). In graphs comparing life expectancy with the percentage of GNP spent on health care in the United States, Lundberg observed that the major gains in life expectancy occurred when health care expenditures were at their lowest (Lundberg 1992, pp. 2521- 2522). Average life expectancy in the U.S. has risen from 49 in 1900 to 77 in 1990. But the major part of this increase (from 49 to 72) occurred before 1960, during a period when the portion of GNP spent on health care was between 3% and 5.5%. This means that the major part of the increase in life expectancy came before the sharp increases in health care expenditures that began in the 1960s. Between 1960 and 1990, as the portion of GNP spent on health care rose from 5.5% to 12.5%, life expectancy rose only from 72 to 77 years.

In a study that sought to determine the impact of medical services on health status, using data for the years 1963 and 1970, Benham and a colleague concluded that "positive increments in non-obstetric medical services for adult population groups from 1963 to 1970 did not lead to improvements of health" (Benham and Benham, 1975b, p. 227). This study is important and not only for the conclusion drawn, but also because part of the data comes from the mid-sixties, a period after Medicaid and Medicare, a kind of decent minimum project, were implemented in the United States.

There is further evidence that current and past expenditures on health care in this country, as well as others, has had little impact on mortality. In making this claim, one must, of course, clearly draw a distinction between "clinical practice on the one hand and the larger responsibilities of medicine as an institution on the other" (McKeown 1979, p. 191). Mckeown, after studying the decline in mortality rates in several countries since the end of the 17th century, concluded that the decline was "due predominantly to a reduction of deaths from infectious diseases" (McKeown 1979, p. 45).

With respect to non-infective diseases as a cause of death in the 18th, 19th, and 20th centuries, McKeown concluded that "the contribution of clinical medicine to the prevention of death and increase in expectation of life in the past three centuries was smaller than that of the other influences" (McKeown 1979, p. 91). McKeown attributes improvement in nutrition as being the most important, while improvements in public hygiene accounted for at least a fifth of the reduction of the death rate between the mid nineteenth and mid twentieth centuries. Vaccinations, with the exception of the smallpox vaccine, "whose contribution was small" (McKeown 1979, p. 78), and medicines made little contribution until sulphonamides were introduced in the mid 1930s. Changes in reproductive practices were also very significant, McKeown argues, for they "ensured that the improvement in health brought about by other means was not reversed by rising numbers" (McKeown 1979, p. 78). In his later study, McKeown reached basically the same conclusion "it is most unlikely that personal medical care had a significant effect on the trend of mortality in the eighteenth and nineteenth centuries" (McKeown 1988, p. 81).

In another recent study of the decline in mortality in the United States since 1900, it was found that the vast majority of the decline occurred before the mid-sixties explosion of health care expenditures, or in the words of the authors of the study:

It is evident that the beginning of the precipitate and still unrestrained rise in medical care expenditures began when nearly all (92 percent) of the modern decline in mortality this century had already occurred.

Markowitz *et al*, argue that the general decline in mortality in the late nineteenth century, which was due to "various sanitary reforms, antitoxins, protective sera and increased education" (Markowitz and Rosner, 1973, p. 88), was responsible in part for the medical reform movement of the era, for physicians were worried that "the actual need for the physician would decline" (Markowitz and Rosner, 1973, p. 88).

Three additional studies also basically concluded the same thing: "For most of history, medical care has been irrelevant in the determination of aggregate social indices whatever comfort it may have brought to particular individuals" (Hartwell 1974, p. 3); and "indeed, from a historical standpoint, nutritional improvement, establishment of sanitary control and the spread of educational achievement in industrialized nations have been clearly more significant for improving the health of nations (particularly in the reduction or postponement of mortality) than medical delivery has been" (Perlman 1974, p. 21); and "the marginal contribution of medical care to life expectancy, holding the state of the art constant, is also very small. Improvements in medical science (primarily new drugs), however, have had significant effects during the period 1930-60" (Fuchs 1974, p. 174).

In addition to these general observations, the leading causes of death in the United States and Canada are causes for which the physician can offer only palliative care, and only after the fact. In both the U.S. and Canada the four leading causes of death, in order, are heart disease, cancer, cerebrovascular diseases (or principally strokes), and accidents (Center for Disease Control, 1992, p. 1450; Crichton *et al*, 1990, p. 16).

A recent Canadian study on the impact of medical care on mortality in Canada, despite almost all of the provinces having had some degree of national health insurance throughout the course of the study, from 1958 to 1988, and despite "spectacular gains in utilization" (Barer and Evans, 1986, p. 83) during the years studied, could only conclude that "medical care probably had an important impact on changes in mortality rates from amenable diseases" (Desmeules and Semenciw, 1991, p. 211, emphasis added).

The evidence presented, while perhaps not conclusive, certainly does give one cause to be skeptical about the institution of medicine's overall contribution to life expectancy and the decline in mortality rates. The source for this skepticism is, as the McKinlay's graph shows, that increasing health care expenditures are not producing proportionate returns. Furthermore, the accumulated evidence suggests that further study of medicine's alleged contribution to the increase in life expectancy is at least warranted. However, even if further investigations did reveal that medicine's overall contribution to increases in life expectancy and decreases in mortality were more than the aforementioned studies suggest, the burden of proof for demonstrating that a universal project of ensuring delivery of health care is better than the current disaggregated means would still rest on Buchanan's shoulders.

Buchanan's arguments if successful, like Daniels' fair equality of opportunity argument, would permit free-riding by those who fail to take care of their health, and for two reasons. First, he provides no mechanism for distinguishing between contributory negligence with respect to becoming sick and/or injured and those who happen to become sick or injured through no fault of their own. Thus, if we did have a basic moral duty of beneficence, as Buchanan has suggested, then given that those who do not contribute to their own morbidity are more deserving and that we have only a limited beneficence budget, Buchanan must show why both groups have an equal claim, or he must draw the distinction we just drew. If the former, then, in addition to the other problems we have argued his argument faces, he must show why beneficence should provide after-the-fact support to people who engage in wilful neglect of their own health. If the latter, he faces similar problems if he wants those who wilfully neglect their own health to be covered under the decent minimum project.

The last response to Buchanan's enforced beneficence argument concerns the empirical data that can be found to suggest that, especially with respect to Americans, people have met their charitable obligations. We grant that this evidence does not touch Buchanan's theoretical argument, although it might at least force Buchanan to address the assumption on which his argument rests.

People do contribute to charity, and in amounts which should be sufficient to meet the demands of the decent minimum project. For example, in a recent telethon, the 1991 Jerry Lewis Telethon for Muscular Dystrophy, over $42 million in voluntary contributions was raised in a three day period. This amount is, by itself, a substantial amount of money. However, when we look at the total of all voluntary charitable donations for a given year the amount is absolutely staggering. In 1988 Americans voluntarily contributed to charity a total of $104.3 billion ("Americans Donated $104 Billion in '88," p. A16)![68] This is $2 billion more than the $102.3 billion the U.S. spent on health care in 1973 (Gibson 1979, p. 22). In fact this amount is equal to 19% of the $546 billion Americans spent on health care in 1988, the year Americans made their $104.3 billion contribution to charity, and 16% of the $666.2 billion they spent on health care in 1990 (Levit *et al*, 1991b, p. 47).

Comparable Canadian figures are unavailable, but nonetheless we can note that Canadian business donated over $75 million in 1988 (Diffy 1990, p. 59). However, not only does this figure not include individual contributions, it may be substantially less than the actual amount Canadian business contributed, for in the study which generated this figure, only 20% of the companies contacted responded to the request for information (Diffy 1990, p. xi). Given the unavailability of comparable Canadian data, we shall focus on the American figure. In addition, we should also note that no other country has as good a history of philanthropy as the United States.

Of the $104.3 billion Americans donated in 1988, $86.7 billion came from individuals; this represents a 7.3% increase from the $80.7 billion donated in 1987. Donations in 1988 from estates totaled $6.7 billion, donations from foundations came to $6.1 billion, while businesses contributed $4.7 billion. In addition one should also not overlook the fact that the total amount donated may have been higher were it not for changes in the American tax laws. It was argued, with respect to the 1986 Tax Reform Act, that some philanthropic contributions were less than what they might have been because the act eliminated charitable deductions for taxpayers who do not itemize. It was also argued that the Tax Reform Act reduced the tax advantage of donating property that appreciated in value ("Americans Donated $104 Billion in '88," p. A16).

The breakdown of recipients of this $104.3 billion is quite interesting as well. Of the $104.3 billion donated, $9.5 billion was specifically donated to health care, while $10.4 billion was given to human services. Donations to the arts, culture, and the humanities came to $6.8 billion, while education received $9.7 billion; $3 billion went to environmental, civil rights, social justice, and women's organizations. The category known simply as "all others" received $16.5 billion; this category included overseas donations.[69]

We quote these figures at length for several reasons. The first reason is that these figures provide empirical evidence which suggests that people may have already met their basic moral duty of charity by contributing almost 20% of 1988 American health care expenditures but without an account of what constitutes a decent minimum we cannot be sure. In fact, the total amount Americans contributed to charity exceeds the amount the General Accounting Office estimated would be necessary to insure the uninsured, $18 billion, and additional services to those already insured, $46 billion, by $40.3 billion (General Accounting Office 1991, p. 7). Furthermore, the total amount contributed by Americans to charity exceeds the $78.2 billion that Shiels and her colleagues estimated would be needed to offset the increase in utilization if the United States adopted a Canadian-style system of health care delivery (Shiels *et al*, 1992, p. 20). However, of the amount donated by Americans, only $9.5 billion was specifically donated to health care. But Americans did donate an additional $10.4 billion to human services. If we assume that this latter category includes health care related concerns, which is likely, then Americans would have donated almost $20 billion to health care and health care related concerns, an amount which exceeds the General Accounting Office estimate of $18 billion needed to insure the uninsured, plus an additional $84.4 billion to non-health related concerns. Surely such generosity meets the "basic moral obligation of charity or beneficence to those in need" (Buchanan 1984, p. 69).

Americans not only voluntarily make charitable contributions, but they also allocate their contributions according to their preferences. Health care is important to most Americans, as evidenced above, but they also have other concerns. These concerns are reflected in the distribution of their voluntary charitable contributions. Hence, it is incumbent upon Buchanan to demonstrate not only why his enforced beneficence argument should be applied to health care as opposed to any of the other concerns listed earlier, but also why the 19% of 1988 American health care expenditures actually contributed is not sufficient for people to have met their basic moral duty of beneficence.

We have examined the empirical evidence of charity, at least in the United States, and while this does little if anything with respect to Buchanan's theoretical point, it does suggest that Americans may be able voluntarily to meet their basic moral duty of beneficence. This, of course, cannot be established until such time as we have some account of what constitutes a decent minimum. Nevertheless, the accumulated weight of the objections we have raised against Buchanan's enforced beneficence arguments are sufficient to conclude that he is unsuccessful in his attempt to establish a positive right to a decent minimum of health care.

Even assuming, with respect to his two enforced beneficence arguments, that people are rational and beneficent, Buchanan could still not show what he needed to show in order for his argument to succeed. It seems that our rationality, even when tempered by a duty of beneficence, may preclude us from being able to accomplish what we acknowledge to be the good without some sort of external mechanism that forces us to do what we believe we ought. But political solutions like enforced beneficence are costly, and in some cases much more costly than either social or moral solutions. Buchanan's external mechanism of enforced beneficence is a possible solution to the assurance problem, but it is not the only solution. In this chapter we have identified an alternative solution to the assurance problem,

Schmidtz's social solution of assurance contracts. There are also moral solutions and in the following chapters we will consider one such moral solution, Gauthier's theory of justice. In the course of explicating Gauthier's theory, we shall attempt to ascertain how well it fares with respect to solving the problem our rationality imposes on us. We shall then apply certain principles of his theory to one of the major problems we have identified in the previous chapters, specifically the issue of rights to health care.

Chapter V

The Foundation for a Just Minimum of Health Care

The main aim of David Gauthier's recent book *Morals By Agreement* is to argue for a "contractarian rationale for morality" (Gauthier 1986, p. 9).[70] As a contractarian, Gauthier, like Rawls, endorses the idea that society is a "cooperative venture for mutual advantage among persons conceived as not taking an interest in one another's interests" (Gauthier 1986, p. 10; Rawls 1971, p. 4 and p. 13).[71] The rationale for agreeing to enter such a society is quite straightforward: a society, "analyzed as a set of institutions, practices, and relationships" (Gauthier 1986, p. 11), that can guarantee for each of its members that each will benefit from entering such a society, as opposed to what each could expect from remaining in a Hobbesian state of nature, is one that is sure to have the voluntary support of its members. If such a society is possible, then it must be the case that there is a set of conditions under which each person would voluntarily agree to enter into such a society.

In Gauthier's case the agreement to enter such a society is a hypothetical agreement, not an actual agreement.[72] Furthermore, the people who are a party to this hypothetical agreement does not include everyone. Gauthier explicitly excludes animals and those who cannot contribute to the cooperative enterprise (Gauthier 1986, p. 268).[73] The people who are party to the hypothetical agreement are highly idealized agents; that is, they are conceived to be rational in the sense that they are concerned to maximize their expected utility and they are fully informed with respect to each other's utility function. In addition, Gauthier assumes that bargaining is cost free.[74]

Gauthier's task, once armed with these assumptions, is four-fold. First, he must tell us what it is that people would agree to with respect to distributing the benefits of cooperation. Second, he must then demonstrate why these highly idealized agents would agree to what he says they would agree to. Third, he must resolve the compliance problem; that is, he must demonstrate why it would be rational for people so conceived to keep their agreement. For, while it may be rational to make an agreement, it may not be rational to comply with the agreement once the conditions under which the original agreement was made change. However, prior to reaching agreement concerning which principle is to govern the distribution of the benefits of cooperation, Gauthier must first specify the initial bargaining position, or with what assets are the bargainers allowed to approach the bargaining table. Unless people reach agreement on what they are entitled to bring to the bargaining table, then either there will be no other agreements or any agreement reached would be unstable.

With respect to the question of what these highly idealized agents would agree to, Gauthier argues that they would agree to distribute the benefits of cooperation according to the principle of minimax relative concession. With respect to the two questions of why they would agree to this principle and why they would comply with their agreements Gauthier argues that they would agree to the principle of minimax relative concession and keep their agreements for doing so would maximize one's expected utility. Finally, Gauthier's solution to the problem of defining the initial bargaining position is the non-cooperative outcome constrained by Gauthier's interpretation of Locke's proviso.

The arguments constructed by Gauthier to reach these conclusions are compelling. In fact, it has been said of Gauthier that he has come "closer to pulling off this 'argument of a lifetime' than anyone could legitimately expect" (Kraus and Coleman, 1987, p. 721). But what is the argument and why is it important? It is the task of this chapter to answer these, as well as some other important questions. We shall begin with Gauthier's solution to the initial bargaining position, the non-cooperative outcome constrained by Gauthier's interpretation of Locke's proviso -- or as we shall now refer to it, Gauthier's proviso -- and Gauthier's derivation of negative rights to one's person and property.

Locke originally conceived of the proviso as one of the conditions that must be satisfied in the state of nature in order for individuals to acquire a negative right to private property. He argued that one could acquire such a negative right provided that there was "enough, and as good left in common for others" Locke, ch. v, para. 33). Nozick, like Locke, was concerned to provide an argument for the original acquisition of property and thus substantiate his entitlement theory of justice. He interpreted Locke's proviso -- that there be enough and as good left in common -- to mean that "the situation of others is not worsened" (Nozick 1974, p. 175).

Given that Gauthier is concerned not merely to provide an argument for a negative right to property but also to provide an argument for the negative right to one's original factor endowments -- that is the natural assets one is born with -- he found Nozick's interpretation of Locke's proviso to be too demanding. He argues that Nozick's interpretation of Locke's proviso may require one to worsen one's own situation so as to avoid worsening the situation of others. Locke held, and Gauthier agrees with him, that preserving one's own life is more important than preserving the life of another. Hence, Gauthier modified Nozick's interpretation of Locke's proviso to allow for one to preserve one's own life. Thus Gauthier interprets Locke's proviso so that it "prohibits bettering one's situation through interaction that worsens the situation of another" (Gauthier 1986, p. 205). An example will help illustrate this.

Imagine a person that is drowning in a lake. Suppose further that his being in the lake came about in either one of two ways. In the first instance I could have pushed him into the lake, and in the second, he could have accidentally fell into the lake. If I pushed him into the lake and then fail to rescue him, I have worsened his situation, for he would have been better off had I been absent. If he accidentally fell into the lake and if I should happen to pass by and, hearing his cries for assistance, ignore them and continue on my way, then, while I may have failed to better his situation, I have not worsened it. I have not worsened his situation, for the outcome he could expect, by my passing by and not saving him, is the same outcome he could expect if I had not come along. Thus, on Gauthier's account, the base point for determining whether one is made better or worse off is determined by the outcome one could expect in the absence of another.

Rational agents, Gauthier argues, would only consider approaching the bargaining table if they knew that what each initially brought to the table had been acquired fairly; that is to say that neither of the players would have been placed at a strategic disadvantage by the coercive efforts of the other. If an initial acquisition was unfair, then the bargaining situation itself would be contaminated such that any outcome would be unfair. This would lead to problems with compliance and hence social instability. But if the prebargaining baseline is the non-cooperative outcome constrained by Gauthier's proviso, then, as no one would have bettered his situation through interaction that worsened the situation of the other, each party could bring to the bargaining table what he could make use of "in the absence of his fellows" (Gauthier 1986, p. 209).

In the absence of his fellows, each person could only make use of his natural factor endowments; that is, his physical and mental capacities. In the drowning example, where the person accidentally fell into the water, in the absence of all others, he could expect to drown. Thus, the first step in Gauthier's derivation of rights is that the non-cooperative outcome, constrained by his proviso, "gives each person [an] exclusive [negative] right to the use of his body and its powers, his physical and mental capacities" (Gauthier 1986, p. 210). The second step in Gauthier's derivation of rights is to show how a person can have a negative right in objects external to himself by extending the liberty he has to use his own powers, as long as such use does not violate Gauthier's proviso. This latter right, at least initially, is not an exclusive right to the possession of the fruits of one's labor, as it was with Locke, but rather it is a negative right in the "effects of one's labor" (Gauthier 1986, p. 211).

Suppose, Gauthier argues, that in the absence of cooperative interaction with another, you cultivate some plot of land. Insofar as your cultivation of the land is independent of cooperative interaction with others, then, even though you may worsen their situation by your preemptive activity of cultivation, you would still not have violated Gauthier's proviso. For, even though you may have worsened the situation of another, your worsening of their situation was not only independent of any cooperative interaction with them, it was also incidental to your bettering your own position.

On the other hand, now suppose that someone seized the product of your labor. Because such a seizure would allow her to better herself at your expense, Gauthier's proviso would be violated. Recall that each person has a negative right to what she can use in the absence of her fellows. But for your presence and your activity of cultivating the land, there would be no product for her to seize. Hence, in seizing it, she betters her situation by worsening yours and Gauthier's proviso is therefore violated.

Gauthier does not conclude from this argument that one thereby has an exclusive positive right to the fruits of one's labor. Rather all that he concludes is that one has a negative right "in the effects of one's labor" (Gauthier 1986, p. 211). He then goes on to allow that one could seize the fruits of another's labor if they paid "full compensation" as opposed to "market compensation" (Gauthier 1986, p. 211). Full compensation is required because it does not leave one with a net loss of utility. If one paid market compensation for the seizure of the fruits of another's labor, then one might better the victim's situation because market compensation sometimes exceeds full compensation. But if Gauthier's proviso requires full compensation for the seizure of the fruits of one's labor, then this means one has the negative right, not to the fruits of one's labor, but rather one has a negative right in the fruits of one's labor. Gauthier then concludes that the migration from a Hobbesian state of nature to a Lockean state of nature is complete.

In a Hobbesian state of nature people have the liberty to use what they can use in the absence of their fellows, their basic natural endowments. In moving from the Hobbesian state of nature to the Lockean state of nature, people gain a negative right in, as opposed to a negative right to, the fruits of their labor, lest Gauthier's proviso be violated. But the argument is not yet complete for Gauthier has yet to show how one can make the transition from a Lockean state of nature to a neo-Lockean state of cooperative interaction.

One can move from a Lockean state of nature (or to use Gauthier's terms, market interaction) to a neo-Lockean state of cooperative interaction, Gauthier argues, if each party to the cooperative interaction internalizes the costs of their respective externalities. In the absence of cooperative interaction each party is free to displace the costs of their respective endeavors without violating Gauthier's proviso. Neither party would violate Gauthier's proviso in displacing their costs, for, until they engage in cooperative interaction, they are not bettering their own respective situations through interaction with one another. Until they engage in actual cooperative interaction they need not internalize the costs of their respective activities for the costs each imposes on the other is not necessary to the benefit each receives from their own independent activity. However, should the parties want to cooperate with each other, then, lest Gauthier's proviso be violated, each must internalize their respective displaced costs. If either party did not internalize his own displaced costs, then he would be bettering his own situation through interaction that worsened the situation of the other, thus violating Gauthier's proviso. Note that we have not yet completely emerged from the Hobbesian state of nature to the Lockean state of nature, nor to a neo-Lockean state of nature. What Gauthier is arguing is that it is a necessary condition for such movements to take place that each person internalize their respective displaced costs. Once such costs have been internalized, Gauthier argues, the parties should be willing to approach the bargaining table. Thus for Gauthier the prebargaining baseline is the non-cooperative outcome constrained by his proviso.

The fourth step in Gauthier's derivation of rights to person and property is to move from a negative right in to a negative right to the fruits of one's labors. This move, if successful, introduces an exclusive negative right to possess property, that is, land and other goods. Suppose Eve were to seek exclusive control over some piece of the commons; that is, an exclusive negative right to the property in question. She justifies her claim on the grounds that not only would her claim not violate Gauthier's proviso, but also on the grounds that the others may be better off. The reasons that the others may be better off are twofold.

First, in seeking an exclusive negative right to some portion of the commons, "Eve proposes to give up her [negative] right in the remaining commons (Gauthier 1986, p. 216). Thus, even though there may be less of the commons remaining after Eve claims her portion, what does remain is shared with less people.

Second, given that Eve puts her claimed-to portion of land to good use, others stand to benefit from her, for they now have an opportunity to engage in mutually beneficial transactions. If the land remained as a commons and there was a sufficiently large population, then not only would there be no opportunity for mutually beneficial transactions, there would also likely be, as David Schmidtz observes, "a mad rush to mutual starvation" (Schmidtz 1991, p. 22). Moreover, as Schmidtz also argues, "until access to the land is restricted, people will have the opportunity and the incentive to overuse it, and some of them as a matter of fact will overuse it, thereby not leaving enough and as good for others" (Schmidtz 1991, p. 23).

If the effects of Eve's exclusive use of a portion of the commons is, as Gauthier has argued, mutually beneficial, then his proviso has not been violated. Eve has not made herself better off by claiming exclusive use to a portion of the commons through interaction that worsened the situation of others. The question that now remains to be answered is, would someone violate Gauthier's proviso by taking the fruits of Eve's labor? On the one hand, if someone took the fruits of Eve's labors, then that person would make himself better off at Eve's expense, thereby violating Gauthier's proviso. On the other hand, if Eve's claimed portion of the commons were returned to the commons, then, Gauthier argues, everyone would be made worse off and, once again, his proviso would be violated and on two counts. First, everyone would be made worse off, for they would now no longer have the opportunity to engage in transactions that were mutually beneficial. Second, the benefits obtained by those who sought to have Eve's claimed portion of the commons returned to the commons would be bettering themselves at the expense of the rest of the community. Therefore, Gauthier concludes, "if [Eve did] not violate [his] proviso by her claim, then anyone subsequently interfering with that claim would violate [his] proviso" and "Eve's [negative] right is thus vindicated" (Gauthier 1986, p. 216).

Gauthier's proviso is not the outcome of rational agreement. "Rather, it is a condition that must be accepted by each person for such agreement to be possible" (Gauthier 1986, p. 16). Negative rights to one's basic endowment and negative rights to property, Gauthier concludes, "provide the starting point for, and not the outcome of, agreement. [Negative rights] are what each person brings to the bargaining table, not what she takes from it" (Gauthier 1986, p. 222).

Once rational agents have agreed on the initial bargaining position, they are then in a position to bargain over the principle that would be used to distribute the benefits of cooperation. Gauthier argues that they would agree to the principle of minimax relative concession. To illustrate the principle of minimax relative concession, let us consider an actual medico-legal case, John Moore *v* The Regents of California (Moore *v* The Regents of California, 1990). We shall first present the facts of the case and then ascertain how Gauthier's principle of minimax relative concession would apply.

Moore, after he learned he had hairy-cell leukemia, became a patient of UCLA Medical Center, under the care of Dr. Golde. Golde confirmed Moore's diagnosis *via* various tests on blood, bone marrow, and other bodily substances. During this time Golde, as well as the other named codefendents, were aware that certain rare blood and body tissues could be exploited for their commercial value, and that having a patient like Moore who could contribute these rare bodily substances would be of great commercial advantage.

On October 8, 1976, Golde obtained Moore's consent for a splenectomy after he, Golde, recommended the operation. On October 20, 1976, unnamed surgeons, not Golde, performed a splenectomy on Moore. However, unbeknownst to Moore, both Golde and Quan, a UCLA researcher, without informing Moore before the operation or before his consent for the operation was obtained, had made arrangements for the commercial exploitation of Moore's rare tissue samples. After the removal of Moore's spleen, Moore returned to the UCLA Medical Center from Seattle several times between 1976 and 1983. Each occasion of Moore's return to UCLA medical Center was at the request of Golde for the expressed purpose of conducting follow-up care and treatment. On each of these occasions more bodily fluids and tissue samples were taken.

Again, unbeknownst to Moore and without his consent, Golde and Quan were continuing their investigations into Moore's unique blood and tissue samples. Subsequently, in August 1979, Golde and Quan managed to establish a cell line from Moore's T-lymphocytes. On January 30, 1981 the UCLA regents applied for a patent on the new cell line and listed Golde and Quan as the inventors (Moore 1990, pp. 148-149). Based on established UCLA policy all involved, except Moore, would enjoy a share of the royalties. The potential amount of money that Golde and Quan's research on Moore's unique blood and tissue sample could earn was substantial; Moore estimated it in the range of $3.01 billion.

For our immediate purposes it is not necessary for us to evaluate this case morally or legally. Our concern is to use this case as an example to illustrate the implications of Gauthier's principle of minimax relative concession. Imagine that, contrary to fact, Moore and Golde both knew that Moore's unique blood and body tissues were extremely rare and that there was a potential to earn substantial economic rewards if the samples were made available to Golde and his research efforts were successful. Imagine further that Golde approaches Moore with an offer to conduct research on the samples of Moore's blood and bodily tissues after completion of the splenectomy. We assume Moore, in virtue of Gauthier's derivation of rights to one's initial endowments, has a negative right to his blood and bodily tissue and that he has the liberty to dispose of it as he sees fit. We ignore here any possible legal or moral quandaries concerning medical research, profiting from the sale or donation of bodily tissue, or any other such complication. Also, lest we be led astray on digressions, we stipulate that Moore needed the operation and would have had the operation, regardless of the pecuniary possibilities.

Suppose Golde tells Moore, and Moore verifies Golde's claims through independent sources, that by cooperating with Golde's research efforts both could earn a substantial amount of money if the research proved successful. Both Moore and Golde are in a unique position, or so we imagine. Golde cannot conduct his research on new cell lines without Moore's cooperation and there is no other researcher with Golde's expertise. Thus if they cooperate, both will benefit. If they do not cooperate, then, given our assumptions, neither will benefit. Moore will have his operation, the tissue samples will be destroyed, and Golde will have to wait for another person with Moore's rare bodily substances to conduct his research.

On the other hand, if they decide to cooperate, then they must decide on some division of the cooperative surplus; that is, the amount remaining after both Moore and Golde subtract their costs. Moore can't conduct the research without the assistance of Golde and therefore, if he cannot find another researcher with Golde's unique talents, he can expect no return from his unique endowment. Golde, on the other hand, has no other source of such rare bodily tissues. Golde, having read Gauthier, and being familiar with the principle of minimax relative concession, tells Moore he will conduct the research on Moore's tissues for a 50% share of the cooperative surplus.

The principle of minimax relative concession is appealed to by both Golde and Moore during the process of reaching an agreement. Both Moore and Golde reason that if there is no agreement, then Moore's tissue will be worthless and there will be no cooperative surplus. If there is agreement, then the cooperative surplus, the resulting sum of the combined contributions of both Moore and Golde, minus their factor costs, will need to be fairly distributed. Minimax relative concession, Gauthier argues, is the principle they would appeal to for distributing the co-operative surplus.

Moore and Golde, as equally rational players, would reason as follows. First, both Moore and Golde would advance their maximal claim; that is, each would claim the entire surplus. Since neither would accept the maximal claim the other made, if they want to reach an agreement, they would then have to make smaller claims. They would continue to make smaller and smaller claims up to the point such that any smaller claim would leave one party with a larger portion of the cooperative surplus. That is to say each reasons that there is a feasible concession point that every rational person is willing to entertain and they minimize their own maximum concession relative to this feasible concession point (Gauthier 1986, pp. 141-143). Once they have reasoned to minimizing their maximum relative concession they can then reach an agreement. Moore and Golde both stand to gain from cooperation. Therefore, they each would minimize their maximum relative concession and reach agreement. In this example, Moore and Golde would each receive 50% of the cooperative surplus. However, this example assumes that both contributed equally to the production of the cooperative surplus. If their contributions to the cooperative surplus were not equal, then the agreement they reached concerning their share of the cooperative surplus would reflect this inequality.

The non-cooperative outcome, constrained by Gauthier's

proviso, is Gauthier's solution to the problem of defining the initial bargaining position. Minimax relative concession is the principle which is to govern the distribution of the benefits of cooperation. This is what people would agree to, or so Gauthier has argued. However, as we stated at the beginning of this chapter, Gauthier not only has to show what people would agree to but also why they would keep their agreements; that is, he has to solve the compliance problem. One reason why rational utility maximizers might be concerned to constrain their behavior, such that they would make and comply with those agreements they have made, is that they might stand to benefit more from keeping their agreements than breaking them.

The compliance problem is best illustrated by the Prisoner's Dilemma. Suppose Golde and Quan conspired to defraud Moore of his rare tissue samples, and they agree that if they should be caught, they will not testify against one another. Both Golde and Quan, as rational utility maximizers, are equally concerned about spending as little time in jail as possible for their misdeeds, notwithstanding their agreement to keep silent should they be caught. Their reasoning is depicted below:

	Quan confesses	Quan does not confess
Golde confesses	5 years each	1 year for Golde
	5 years each	10 years for Quan
Golde does not confess	10 years for Golde	2 years each
	1 year for Quan	

The dilemma they face is that if they both confess, they each get five years. If one confesses, and the other does not, then the one who confesses only gets one year, while the other gets ten. If neither confesses, which was what they agreed upon, then they get two years each. While this latter outcome may be the best outcome for both of them, they each have an incentive to confess. As equally rational utility maximizers, they are both concerned to spend as little time in jail as possible, regardless of what happens to the other. Thus, they both confess, for they cannot rely upon the other not to, and they both spend five years in jail. Had they been able to keep their agreement not to confess, they would have had to spend only two years in jail.

To solve the compliance problem Gauthier makes a distinction between those actors who are straightforward maximizers of utility (SMs) and those who are constrained maximizers of utility (CMs). A CM is a person who is "disposed to comply with mutually advantageous moral constraints, provided he expects similar compliance from others" (Gauthier 1986, p. 15), while an SM is a person who is disposed to straightforwardly maximize his utility on each occasion. Gauthier then argues that a rational agent would choose, given the alternatives of either adopting an SM disposition or a CM disposition, to adopt constrained maximization as his disposition for strategic interaction.

It is important to note here that Gauthier makes a move that others involved with game theory have not made. The received view among game theorists is that one identifies rationality at the level of particular choices. Thus on the received view a choice would be rational if and only if it maximized the actor's expected utility on that particular occasion. But on Gauthier's view choice involves dispositions. He says,

> We identify rationality with utility maximization at the level of dispositions to choose. A disposition is rational if and only if an actor holding it can expect his choices to yield no less utility than the choices he would make were he to hold any alternative disposition (Gauthier 1986, pp. 182-183).

This move is important for Gauthier, for it allows him to resolve the compliance problem. Gauthier argues that adopting either a CM disposition or an SM disposition affects the situations one could reasonably expect to find oneself in. He then argues that CMs will fare better than SMs.

> A straightforward maximizer, who is disposed to make maximizing choices, must expect to be excluded from cooperative arrangements which he would find advantageous. A constrained maximizer may expect to be included in such arrangements. She benefits from her disposition, not in the choices she makes, but in her opportunities to choose (Gauthier 1986, p. 183).

There is an additional characteristic of CMs that Gauthier argues for to support his conclusion that choosing a disposition of constrained maximization yields a greater expected utility than choosing a disposition of straightforwardly maximizing utility. CMs (and SMs) are "translucent" as opposed to being either "transparent" or "opaque." To say that persons are translucent is to say that we can ascertain their disposition to cooperate or not cooperate, "not with certainty, but as more than mere guesswork" (Gauthier 1986, p. 174). If persons were transparent, then we could ascertain their disposition with certainty; if persons were opaque, then ascertaining their disposition would be mere guesswork. Gauthier rejects transparency in favor of translucency because his argument in favor of a CM disposition would have little practical import in the real world if he only managed to show this given the idealizing assumption that all persons were transparent. Gauthier thinks that people really are, to some degree, translucent and this, he argues, helps to tie his ideal argument to the real world.

Gauthier also argues that CMs would be "narrowly compliant" as opposed to being "broadly compliant." A narrowly compliant person is one "who is disposed to cooperate in ways that, followed by all, yield nearly optimal and fair outcomes," and a person who is broadly compliant is a person who is disposed to cooperate in ways that, followed by all, "merely yield her some benefit in relation to universal non-compliance" (Gauthier 1986, p. 178).

We should now be able to see how Golde and Quan can obtain the Pareto-optimal outcome; that is, only serving two years. If both Golde and Quan were narrowly compliant and reasonably translucent CMs, then they would have agreed not to confess should they ever happen to find themselves in a Prisoner's Dilemma. Because they were CMs, (CMs who were narrowly compliant and reasonably translucent), and not SMs, they could expect that the other would not confess by virtue of their each having chosen the disposition to be a constrained maximizer. If they were both SMs, then they would not expect the other to cooperate under these circumstances.

This is the essence of Gauthier's argument for morals by agreement, or at least those aspects which concern us, with some of the particular details omitted. Gauthier's contractarian rationale for morality is not without its difficulties. It is, however, an important work in moral theory. If Gauthier's argument is sound, then we might no longer require a political solution like Buchanan's or a social solution like Schmidtz's for some of our more intractable social problems; the justification for many, if not all of our social programs and policies, would be questionable. If Gauthier's argument is successful, we would be compelled by the logic of his reasoning to accept his conclusions on a new moral order.

Our task in the next chapter is to ascertain whether or not Gauthier's theory of justice, his new moral order, would endorse some sort of positive right to health care, and if so, what kind? In the course of determining whether Gauthier's theory of justice can endorse a positive right to health care, we shall have cause to consider Arrow's justification for the social policy of granting the medical profession a monopoly on the practice of health care.

Chapter VI
A Just Minimum of Health Care

Thus far we have covered much ground, both conceptual and empirical, from the comparative analysis of Canada's and the U.S.'s health care systems to the multiple concerns health care consumers have. In addition to the rising costs of health care in Canada and especially in the United States, as well as the increasing number of underinsured and uninsured in the United States, there is concern about the amount of unnecessary and inappropriate care, the incidence of iatrogenic injuries, and both the amount and cost of nosocomial infections. There is also concern about physician-induced demand for medical care, the amount and cost of medical fraud, the problem of self-referral and physician ownership of medical diagnostic and therapeutic centers and equipment. It is within the context of these concerns that the question of justice in health care arises.

In addition, we have considered two alternative approaches to justice in health care, those of Norman Daniels and Allen Buchanan, and found those approaches lacking in several respects. The lessons learned from those two investigations were several. With respect to Daniels' fair equality of opportunity argument for justice in health care, we discovered that attempting to tie health care to a principle of justice that guarantees fair equality of opportunity results in, paradoxically, a decrease in the scope of one's opportunity range. We also discovered not only that the theory-dependent version of the bottomless pit problem was genuine, but also what it was about the bottomless pit problem that made the problem difficult to resolve, namely the morbidity, the supply, and the cost/benefit problems. In order to resolve the theory-dependent version of the bottomless pit problem, we argued, a theory of justice in health care must provide some means from within the theory to constrain the consumption of health care. And finally, with respect to Daniels' argument, we discovered that people have health care wants and desires as well as health care needs, and that these wants and desires are important independently of the Daniels-cum-Boorse biomedical model of disease.

The lessons learned from our investigation of Buchanan's contribution were important as well. In addition to providing the empirical evidence which suggests that Americans may have met their basic moral duty of beneficence to provide a decent minimum of health care, we raised the question of medicine's overall contribution -- as opposed to the actual contribution of individual clinicians to particular patients -- to the health of the citizens of a nation. And while these two general observations did not speak to Buchanan's theoretical point, we were able, nonetheless, to demonstrate that his enforced beneficence arguments failed, and therefore his arguments were unable to provide the needed support for Daniels' argument's admitted weakness. But perhaps the most significant lesson learned was that an instrumental conception of rationality, even though tempered by a duty of beneficence, can make it extremely difficult for people so conceived to achieve what they think they ought.

Our point of departure in this chapter, is Gauthier's theory of morals by agreement. In the previous chapter we explicated Gauthier's derivation of rights, his interpretation of Locke's proviso, and the principle of minimax relative concession. In this chapter we shall advance and defend our main thesis; that is, if the health care delivery systems in Canada and the United States are as the evidence from earlier chapters indicates, then there are certain normative implications which follow from Gauthier's theory of justice. The most notable implication is that people are entitled to a just minimum of health care, or so we shall argue. In support of this thesis, we shall advance two main arguments. We shall first argue that the existing systems of health care delivery in Canada and the United States violates Gauthier's proviso and therefore people whose rights are violated or whose liberties are unjustifiably restricted are owed market compensation for these transgressions. We shall then argue that rational bargainers would not agree to either the Canadian or American system of health care delivery.

The implications of our argument for a just minimum of health care are profound for both countries. While both the Canadian and the American systems of health care delivery violate Gauthier's interpretation of Locke's proviso, they do so for different reasons; consequently the implications for each system of health care delivery are different. In our final chapter, we shall assess the implications of our argument for both countries. In addition, we shall also demonstrate how our argument will allow us to resolve the theory-dependent version of the bottomless pit problem, as well as avoid the other difficulties faced by Daniels' fair equality of opportunity argument and Buchanan's enforced beneficence arguments for a decent minimum of health care.

The concept of health care covers a wide array of goods, services, and people: from the demeanor of nurses to the bedside manner of practicing physicians; from the technical expertise of X-ray and other technicians to the diagnosis and treatments administered by physicians; from the drugs created by the pharmaceutical companies to the prosthetic devices manufactured by other allied businesses. In the United States the amount of money spent on health care in 1988 was $496.6 billion, or 11.2.% of the GNP; in Canada in 1988, $50.4 billion, or 8.7% of the GNP. The question of justice in health care is, however, not just concerned with monetary expenditures, the respective conduct of nurses, doctors, and other paramedical technicians and businesses to the consumer of health care, the patient. Nor is it just concerned with the issue of rights to health care. It is also concerned with, among other things, access to and the cost of these many goods and services, the relationship between each of the participants, and what to do in the case of competing interests, needs, wants, rights, and liberties.

While a person's rights may be violated, a person's liberties may be restricted and the restriction may be either justified or unjustified. If a person's liberties are restricted and if the justification for restricting that person's liberties fails to satisfy Gauthier's proviso, then the liberty-restriction is unjustified. If the liberty-restriction does not violate Gauthier's proviso, then it is justified. Under Gauthier's theory of justice people who have their liberty unjustifiably restricted are owed compensation (Gauthier 1986, pp. 212-216).

There are several justifications that have been advanced in order to justify the restriction of people's liberty. For example, there is Mill's harm principle. Mill says that we may justifiably allow the restriction of one's liberties in order to prevent that person from harming another (Mill 1992, p. 14). The other justifications that have been advanced in order to justify the restriction of people's liberty are the offense principle, the principles of weak and strong paternalism, the principle of legal moralism, and the social welfare principle. Each of these liberty restricting principles attempts to justify the restriction of liberty on different grounds. The offense principle says we are justified in restricting someone's liberty in order to prevent someone from offending others; the principles of weak and strong paternalism attempt to justify the restriction of someone's liberty, respectively, in order to prevent someone from harming himself, or in order to benefit the person whose liberty is restricted. The principle of legal moralism says we are justified in restricting someone's liberty to prevent that person from acting immorally, while the social welfare principle justifies the restriction of liberty in order that others may benefit. But these liberty-restricting principles are not as easily justified as the harm principle and therefore are more controversial than the harm principle. Furthermore, restricting someone's liberty in order to prevent that person from harming another is not in violation of Gauthier's proviso, whereas the other liberty-restricting principles are. Harming someone is worsening their situation and therefore in direct violation of Gauthier's proviso. Recall that the base point for determining whether or not one's situation has been worsened is determined by what you could expect in my absence (Gauthier 1986, p. 204). In my absence, you would not be harmed by me and therefore if I harm you, you are worse off than what you would be in my absence. Hence, Gauthier's proviso sanctions the harm principle. If restricting someone's liberty in order to prevent one person from harming another is not in violation of Gauthier's proviso, then no compensation need be paid to the person whose liberty was thus restricted.

However, suppose we restrict someone's liberty, not to prevent them from harming someone, but rather so that some other person will benefit. Would such a restriction of liberty be in violation of Gauthier's proviso? If so, then compensation must be paid to the person whose liberty was restricted. If not, then compensation is unnecessary. For example, consider the social welfare principle. The social welfare principle says that we are justified in restricting one's liberty in order to benefit others. If my liberty is restricted so that others may benefit, then I am worse off than what I would be in the absence of these others and therefore Gauthier's proviso is violated. If Gauthier's proviso is violated, then, in order to rectify the injustice, I deserve to be compensated.

Under Gauthier's theory of justice, if one's rights have been violated or one's liberties have been unjustifiably restricted, and if either the rights-violation or the liberty-restriction is in violation of his proviso, then one must be given market, rather than full compensation. One must be given market rather than full compensation, for full compensation may be less than what one could have obtained through voluntary exchange. If one only paid full compensation, when full compensation was less than market compensation, then Gauthier's proviso would be violated; that is, the rights-violator would have benefitted himself by worsening the situation of the person whose rights were violated. However, if full compensation is greater than market compensation, as it sometimes is, then full compensation must be paid. For, if full compensation is not paid, then, again, the malefactor would be benefitting himself by worsening the other's situation and Gauthier's proviso would be violated.

For example, suppose you restrict my liberty to engage in voluntary cooperation with another and suppose further that you restrict my liberty with the intention of compensating me for my loss. If you only gave me full compensation for my loss, and the amount of this compensation was less than what I could have received by engaging in voluntary cooperation with another, then I have been made worse off than what I would have been in the absence of your restricting my liberty. You would have violated Gauthier's proviso. However, if you paid me market compensation, what I would have received had I cooperated with the other person, then I would be as well off as I could have been had my liberty not been restricted. In other words, if you do not pay me market compensation, then I am precluded from receiving any part of the benefits you obtained from restricting my liberty.

That people have rights and liberties and that these rights and/or liberties, should they be violated or unjustifiably restricted, require market compensation is important in determining what constitutes justice in health care. But justice in health care need not, at least according to morals by agreement, guarantee a positive right to health care. However, while justice in health care under Gauthier's theory of morals by agreement need not guarantee a positive right to health care, it may in fact do so. Prior to determining how such a right might be guaranteed we must first consider what Gauthier's conception of essential justice demands with respect to people having the liberty to engage in fully voluntary cooperation.

Under Gauthier's theory of morals by agreement people have a negative right to their person and property; that is, they are morally entitled to their initial factor endowments and whatever property they obtained that was not in violation of his proviso. Moreover, people are entitled to the full exercise of their liberty insofar as they are not under a duty to refrain from performing some particular action; that is, they are entitled to engage in any action that is not prohibited by his proviso. If people are entitled to exercise their liberty, then they are entitled to care for their own health to the best of their knowledge and ability; that is, insofar as they do not violate Gauthier's proviso. They are also entitled, provided that Gauthier's proviso does not prohibit it, to seek out others to assist them in caring for their own health.

As things now stand in both Canada and the United States people are allowed under certain conditions to exercise their liberty to care for their own health. They can, among other things, educate themselves and implement any preventive measures not specifically prohibited. Thus one can eat properly, get the proper amount of rest and exercise, refrain from smoking and drinking or only doing so in moderation. As we discussed in Chapter III, preventive measures can accomplish a great deal with respect to ensuring good health. However, people are prevented from doing even the most minor things once they are ill or injured.

For example, and for the most part, if one is suffering from even a minor infection, one cannot purchase the requisite medication to treat the infection, without first obtaining a prescription from a licensed physician. The cost of this prohibition is expensive. One study argued that if penicillin, "one of the least toxic drugs" (Temin 1983, p. 201), was changed from a prescribed drug to an over-the-counter drug, in the United States the "savings to consumers [in 1981 alone] could be over a billion dollars" (Temin 1983, p. 199). The monetary savings to consumers is not the only benefit consumers would reap if penicillin was changed to an over-the-counter drug. If penicillin, and today's generic counterparts, were available as over-the-counter drugs, then people would reap savings not only in terms of the number of visits to their medical practitioner, but also with respect to the knowledge they could acquire and use to treat future minor infections.

The importance of this latter effect should also not be underestimated, For, as studies have shown, "90% of patient contacts with the health care system are for the management of chronic conditions" (Barnhill 1992, p. 43). Of course, not all chronic medical conditions require the use of antibiotics, but that is not the point. The point is that most of patient contacts with the health care system are for the management of chronic conditions. One should note that this 90% figure is in accord with other sets of figures, one of which was cited earlier: that is, only 11.5% of the population is hospitalized each year and 15% of those hospitalized consume some 55% of hospital expenditures (Gagner 1992c, p. 26). In addition, as health-economist Uwe Reinhardt also observes, "in any given year, some 70 to 80% of health care expenditures tend to be caused by only about 10% of the population (Reinhardt 1987, p. 169). And, as Canadian and American demographers inform us, the population will age as the baby boom generation begins to retire in the next fifteen to twenty years. An aging population will only reinforce the veracity of these figures, for the elderly consume a disproportionate amount of health care expenditures (Daniels 1988). While these figures may be interesting, there is additional evidence that physicians are not nearly as necessary for medical care as we once might have thought.

Several recent studies in the United States have demonstrated that some non-physician health professionals, specifically nurse practitioners and physician assistants, can make significant contributions to providing medical care. In analyzing seventeen studies of nurse practitioners and physician assistants that had been conducted in the United States from the mid-1960s to 1980, the authors found that 80% of office visits for adult care and 90% of office visits for pediatric care could safely be delegated to nurse practitioners and/or physician assistants (Record *et al*, 1980, p. 478). The quality of care actually provided by these non-physician health professionals was found to be "at least as high as the care rendered by physicians" (Robyn and Hadley, 1980, p. 450) and patients were just as satisfied with the care received from nurse practitioners and physician assistants as they were with a physicians' care (Robyn and Hadley, 1980, p. 450).

The medical profession unjustifiably restricts people's liberty to care for their own health and well being in numerous other ways as well: a woman who wants birth control pills must also have a prescription; people who want chest x-rays and other routine diagnostic tests, whether for employment purposes, preventive measures, or otherwise, must also first see a physician; the diabetic must routinely seek out a physician to receive a prescription for his daily dose of insulin. The physician does little more than prescribe the requisite medication and/or order the requisite test and communicate the results to the patient or his employer. It is true that the physician assumes some liability for the diagnostic test and procedures he orders. But this liability need not be passed to the physician. The patient could assume the liability -- at least he would not be in violation of Gauthier's proviso if he did -- or he could have the physician or some other consenting third party assume the liability. People who suffer from chronic ailments, like the diabetic, must also see a physician prior to getting the treatment or drugs they already know they need; people who want to see a medical specialist must first go through their own physician to get a referral. The point of these examples, and one could cite numerous others, is not that we do not need physicians at all, for we do, but rather that we do not necessarily need physicians for most of our health care needs and wants. If we were allowed to benefit from medical knowledge acquired during the course of our life, we could use such knowledge to lower the cost of our health care expenditures.

If we had a free market in health care, then not only could non-physician health professionals compete with physicians for patients, but also individuals could exercise their liberty to diagnose and treat themselves or seek out other perhaps less-qualified professionals. This need not seem as far-fetched as it once might have, especially in the light of the study on non-physician practitioners of health care. If 80% of adult office visits and 90% of pediatric office visits can be safely delegated to non-physician practitioners, then, ceterus paribus, we could expect to see a definitive decline in health care costs.

However, while some might concede that some non-physician health professionals could indeed provide some basic level of medical care, most would hesitate at the thought of individuals diagnosing and treating themselves. Be this as it may, it should not detract from the theoretical point which is being made; that is, in a free market in health care individuals would be free to exercise their liberty to diagnose and to treat themselves. People have no moral obligation to refrain from exercising their liberty to diagnose and treat themselves, or to seek out others to assist them in diagnosing and treating themselves; that is, someone who exercises his liberty to care for his own health is not in violation of Gauthier's proviso. However, if one's liberty to care for one's own health is unjustifiably restricted, given that that person has no moral obligation to refrain from exercising his liberty to care for his own health, then Gauthier's proviso has been violated. Gauthier's proviso has been violated, for the person whose liberty has been unjustifiably restricted is worse off than what he would have been in the absence of the unjustified restriction of his liberty and is therefore owed market compensation.

Furthermore, on reflection, this latter idea of individuals diagnosing and treating themselves need not, at least in this day and age, seem as repugnant as it once might have. Individuals today have a much higher basic level of education when it comes to health care than was the case only a few short decades ago. The media has contributed to this general advance in health care education by popularizing a significant portion of the increasing fund of medical knowledge, thus making it accessible to a public whose rising educational level permits many people to comprehend it, at least in its main outline (Haug 1988, p. 50). In addition, the role of computer technology should also not be underestimated. The number of people who are computer literate is increasing and if, as some have argued, medical care is "almost as much a market for information as it is for specific services"

(Pauly 1988, p. 228), then, as we noted earlier, the time may not be too far off when the main issue will not be who has the medical knowledge, but rather who knows how to extract it from its digital storage place (Haug 1988, p. 51). We have already presented evidence that computer programs have been shown to be more accurate than physicians in diagnosing heart attack patients (Waldholz 1991, p. A7). In addition, we mentioned the existence of several different computer programs that are currently being used to diagnose other disease conditions, educate medical and paramedical personnel in anatomy, physiology, pathophysiology, and surgery, and to predict patient outcomes. We also noted that information on the side effects, indications, and contraindications of both prescription and non-prescription drugs is available in digital format. However, we observed that the American Medical Association has advanced the position that marketing such software directly to health care consumers might be in violation of medical licensing laws. It is curious why a professional organization would be opposed to the transmission of information that could be used by consumers of health care to improve their knowledge concerning their health.

In addition to these software programs and other potential sources of medical information, there is also the INTERNET, a world-wide complex of computer networks for exchanging information. The resources available on the INTERNET are vast and cover virtually all areas of interest. For those who need medical information, it is freely available on the INTERNET via the Cleveland Free-net. The Cleveland Free-Net, which started in 1984 as a computer bulletin board system, allows access to any user to ask a medically related question. The questions are answered by physicians and usually within twenty-four hours.

One could object to the above arguments by arguing that even if someone is computer literate, it doesn't follow that that person will also have medical knowledge. Thus, even if one could access the available information, whether by computers or by reading it in a book, this may not be sufficient for one to diagnose and/or treat one's self. This objection is premised on the fact that most medical information is expressed in a technical language that is for the most part inaccessible to the uninitiated. However, this is not an insurmountable obstacle, for most if not all technical language can be translated so that most people can understand it. Thus, while one may at first be perplexed when first encountering terms such as hypertension, hypoglycemic, and tachy-cardia, the confusion disappears when these terms are translated into their functionally equivalent expressions, high blood pressure, low blood sugar, and an excessively rapid heart beat. The translation of technical language into lay terms is easily facilitated with the use of online dictionaries.

We grant *ad arguendo* that most people would not take the time to learn and/or translate the most esoteric medical terms. They might, however, learn enough medical terminology to facilitate the diagnosis and treatment of the numerous minor ailments they are most likely to suffer from. In addition, those who suffer from chronic conditions, if they were allowed to make use of their knowledge to lower their medical costs, would have an incentive to learn as much as they could about their particular ailments. Furthermore, even if most people would not take the time and effort to learn what they needed to know in order to diagnose and/or treat themselves for minor illnesses, some would and in a free market for health care they would be free to do so. More importantly, they would not violate Gauthier's proviso by doing so. Finally, even if some or even most medically-related software programs are not yet sophisticated enough to render your next visit to a physician otiose, they soon will be.

If we require of everyone that they must first see a physician prior to obtaining any health related test, treatment, and/or procedure, then this is not only expensive but also it precludes the individual from being able to take steps to lower his own health care related costs by preventing him from taking advantage of any knowledge he may have acquired from previous experience. This is especially important given that 90% of patient contacts with the health care system are for the management of chronic medical conditions. Furthermore, not only is it the case that most of the more routine diagnostic tests, procedures, and treatments are not only done by para-medical people, nurses, technicians, *et al*, but also the body of knowledge required for assessing the results of these tests, procedures, and treatments is now so standardized that it is readily available to those who take the time and effort to look it up in the appropriate manual, or extract it from its digital storage place.

Some may object that the initial cost of acquiring the information necessary to diagnose and/or treat one's self may be too expensive. After all, medical books cost from $30 to $60 and computer programs typically cost about $100. This objection fails to note that while the initial cost of educating one's self may be high, this cost can be offset by the savings one achieves from not having to go to a physician each and every time one has a minor illness. If people were allowed to freely use the medical knowledge they acquired to lower their health care costs, as they are allowed to use other knowledge to lower their costs in other areas of their lives, then they would have an incentive to acquire such knowledge. We suspect that one of the main reasons why people do not take the opportunity to educate themselves is that, at present, they are prohibited from using such knowledge. If the barriers to using such knowledge were removed, then the demand for such knowledge would increase. The supply of sources to meet that demand would increase as well, thereby lowering one's acquisition costs.

While the existing economic systems of health care delivery in both Canada and the United States might not be a free market *per se*, many barriers to a free market in health care ought to be removed in order to allow people to exercise their liberty to care for their own health. The reason that barriers to a free market in health ought to be removed is that they prohibit people from exercising their liberty to care for their own health, or to seek out other qualified non-physician practitioners, and therefore such barriers are in violation of Gauthier's proviso.

In determining what this violation of Gauthier's proviso might mean with respect to the health care industry, we must consider further how and why the current market in health care differs from a health care market in which there were no barriers or obstacles to the exercising of one's liberty to care for one's own health. The social, economic, and political history of the current health care market in the United States has been traced by Starr (1982), Brown (1979), Markowitz and Rosner (1973), and Hamowy (1979), and in Canada by Hamowy (1984). We need not concern ourselves with all the particular details of these respective historical studies. What should and will concern us are the general conclusions drawn by all, for they highlight not only how the current systems of health care delivery in both Canada and the United States deviates from what would take place under a barrier-free market of health care delivery, but also how and why these deviations occurred. The principal conclusion drawn by all of these authors is that in both countries the respective professional organizations, the AMA and the CMA, systematically sought to increase the political power, the social prestige, and the economic welfare of their organizations as a whole, and their members in particular. The means they employed to accomplish these goals were several: they began by first placing controls on who could legitimately practice medicine by limiting the number of medical schools and restricting admission to those schools. They imposed not only licensing requirements on those who would practice medicine, but also a ban on both competitive advertising and price competition. In order to prevent organized resistance to these actions from those who were to be excluded from the favors these new barriers to free and competitive activity would sanction, they adopted grandfather clauses which included specific competitors. They sought and gained political and legal recognition as a professional body, thereby allowing the medical profession to determine what was and what was not properly within the domain of medicine. With respect to the state delegated power of the AMA to regulate the medical profession, Reuben Kessel has remarked that this "is on par with giving the American Iron and Steel Institute the power to determine the output of steel" (Kessel 1975, p. 280).

The medical profession also unilaterally adopted the practice of what economists call price discrimination, i.e., the scaling of fees to the incomes of particular individual patients; and finally, they advanced moral arguments to the effect that the medical profession was concerned, not with its own welfare, economic or otherwise, but rather the welfare of society in general and their patients in particular. Our main concern in noting these several factors is that it is these very factors which preclude a barrier-free market in the delivery of health care services, thereby preventing people from exercising their liberty to care for their own health or seeking out non-physician practitioners to assist them in meeting their health care needs. More importantly, however, these barriers to a free market in health care delivery are in violation of Gauthier's proviso.

There are other alternative accounts for the aforementioned deviations from a free market in health care delivery. Kenneth Arrow can be read as attempting to justify deviations from a free market in health care insurance by arguing that the free market in health care insurance fails owing to externality problems. The root cause of this market failure, Arrow argues, is "the prevalence of uncertainty" with respect to "the incidence of disease and the efficacy of treatment" (Arrow 1963, pp. 946 and 941 respectively). Uncertainty, in this context, occurs when there are situations where you don't know the probabilities attached to outcomes, because a) you are ignorant or b) there are none. What Arrow means by uncertainty is the ignorance one is faced with concerning the probability that one will be afflicted with a particular disease and the probability that one will receive a treatment that is efficacious with respect to curing the disease.

Arrow lists the following "special structural characteristics" of the medical-care market that the "prevalence of uncertainty" has given rise to: a) irregular and unpredictable demand for health care, b) the expected behavior of the physician, c) uncertainty of the product, d) the restriction of supply, and e) the pricing practices of the medical profession (Arrow 1963, pp. 948-954). If we compared the health care insurance market in the United State to what might be found in a perfectly competitive market, the most notable difference would be that in the latter insurance policies would exist for all conceivable risks. The risks involved in health care are, as Arrow correctly notes, the uncertainty associated with the incidence of disease and the efficacy of treatment. In a perfectly competitive market, people would be able to insure themselves against these risks and would do so if they were sufficiently risk averse and if they could purchase the policy at an actuarially fair price. Given the failure of actual markets to meet the demand for insurance against these risks, we have Pareto-inefficiency; that is, some people could be made better off without making any other person worse off. Given the problem of market failure in health care insurance, Arrow draws two main normative conclusions. The first conclusion Arrow draws is that

> the welfare case for insurance policies of all sorts is overwhelming. It follows that the government should undertake insurance in those case where this market, for whatever reason, has failed to emerge" (Arrow 1963, p. 961; also see Lees and Rice (1965)).

The second conclusion drawn by Arrow is that other social organizations or institutions, in this case the medical profession, may take it upon themselves to correct the market's failure to meet the demand for insurance against these risks (Arrow 1965,

p. 156). Thus, Arrow's normative justification for the existing system of health care delivery is different from the descriptive explanations offered by Starr, Brown, *et al.* While the latter argued that the medical profession's existing monopoly on the practice and delivery of medicine could be explained in terms of the resulting social prestige, political power, and economic welfare of the profession's members, Arrow's normative justification of the medical profession's "special structural characteristics," or non-market system of medical services, is that the medical profession's existing monopoly can be viewed simply as an attempt to solve the market's failure to meet the demand for insurance against such risks.

There is a certain similarity between Arrow's normative justification of a non-market system for medical services and Gauthier's argument for morality. The similarity is that both Arrow and Gauthier argue that markets fail due to externality problems. Their solutions to the problem of market failure, however, are different. While Arrow favors state restrictions on markets when they fail, Gauthier favors moral restrictions. Given these two different solutions to the problem of market failure, the question arises as to why we should prefer one solution rather than the other.

There are several reasons why we ought to prefer Gauthier's to Arrow's solution. However, before we offer these reasons, we must note the difference between Arrow's theoretical solution to the problem of market failure and the presently existing health care institutions. Arrow has argued that either the government should intervene in the case of such market failures or that other social organizations or institutions might take it upon themselves to correct such market failures. In the latter case, Arrow identified some "special structural characteristics" of the medical care market that would mitigate the market failure problem: the expected behavior of the physician, the restriction of supply, and the pricing practices of the medical profession. Given these special structural characteristics and their theoretical efficacy, Arrow's latter solution to the market failure problem would resolve the difficulty. However, as the evidence of earlier chapters was meant to show, the members of the medical profession have not lived up to their expected behavior. They were expected to cooperate in such a manner that they would mitigate the damage of such market failures but have not managed to do so, notwithstanding the profession's own institutional arrangements for ensuring compliance with their expected behavior. Thus, by failing to live up to their expected behavior, they have undermined the very institutions which Arrow thought would be justified because of the market failure problem.

The evidence of the medical profession's failure to comply with their own institutional arrangements for ensuring compliance is overwhelming. Not only have health care costs been steadily rising in both countries, but in the United States there are some 35 million people without health insurance. In addition to these concerns, we also noted the incidence of medical fraud, unnecessary and inappropriate care, the problem of self-referral and physician ownership of medical treatment and diagnostic centers, the incidence of iatrogenic injuries, the amount and cost of nosocomial infections, the problem of physician-induced demand for medical care and the consequent lack of informed consent to unnecessary medical treatments and procedures.

The main reason we ought to prefer Gauthier's solution to Arrow's solution is that Gauthier's solution has the means to ensure compliance with expected behavior; that is, under Gauthier's theory rational agents would not only cooperate, thereby making agreements, but they would also keep their agreements. They would both make and keep their agreements, Gauthier argued, because they would maximize their expected utility by doing so. Theoretically, Arrow's solution would also have rational agents making and keeping their agreements. However, in Arrow's case, the mechanism for ensuring compliance is not internal -- as it is in Gauthier's case -- but rather external; that is, the social organizations and/or institutions would police themselves to ensure that their members would live up to their expected behavior. The empirical evidence, however, demonstrates that these institutions have been unable to ensure the necessary compliance.

Gauthier's solution to the problem of market failure also provides a principled means by which the benefits of cooperation are distributed, minimax relative concession; Arrow's solution does not. Moreover, Gauthier's principle of minimax relative concession is a distributional principle, not a redistributional principle. With Arrow's solution, not only is it the case that there is no principled means by which one can be assured of or guaranteed a share of the benefits of cooperation, but also

Arrow's solution requires a compulsory redistribution from either (or both) the relatively healthy and/or wealthy to the unhealthy and/or poor. That Arrow's solution requires a redistribution of benefits, and not simply a distribution of benefits, is important for it entails that some people will benefit at the expense of others. In other words, a redistribution of benefits would, in effect, sanction free-riding and thus be in violation of Gauthier's proviso. It makes some better off, the relatively unhealthy and/or the poor, by making others worse off, the relatively healthy and/or wealthy.

In addition to these reasons there are other compelling reasons for preferring Gauthier's theory, not Arrow's solution, to the problems of market failure, the most notable of which is that any practical implementation of Arrow's solution rests on empirical data which is at best suspect. For example, if we view the existing system of health care delivery as a practical implementation of Arrow's theoretical solution to the problem of market failure, then we can see how any such implementation must rest on assuming that there is an asymmetry of information problem between the knowledge the physician has and the knowledge her patient has which is sufficient to warrant the implementation of the liberty-restricting principle of weak paternalism. The principle of weak paternalism maintains that we are justified in restricting people's liberty so that people will not harm themselves. When this principle is conjoined with the asymmetry of information problem, it is typically argued that the knowledge base required to understand sufficiently the complexities of modern medicine is simply too great for the average person to comprehend, especially when they are ill, and therefore we are justified in restricting their liberty to decide for themselves what constitutes efficacious medical care. We grant for the sake of argument that if one is seriously ill, then there may indeed be a problem with understanding the complexities of modern medicine. However, even if we grant this assumption, it is still not the case that the majority of doctor/patient encounters involve serious illnesses.

We noted earlier that 80% and 90% of adult and pediatric care could be safely delegated to non-physician practitioners and that 90% of patient contacts with the health care system are for the management of chronic medical conditions. This latter figure, it was suggested, helps explain why such a large percentage of medical care can be safely delegated to non-physician practitioners. In addition, not all health care is a life or death matter. In fact, the vast majority of health care services provided by the medical profession deal with the routine diagnosis and treatment of rather minor illnesses and injuries, which is another reason why such a large percentage of office visits could be safely delegated to non-physician practitioners. Moreover, in both the U.S. and Canada the four leading causes of death, in order, are heart disease, cancer, cerebrovascular diseases (or principally strokes), and accidents (Center for Disease Control, 1992, p. 1450; Crichton *et al*, 1990, p. 16). Not only is it the case that there is little that can be done medically with respect to these leading causes of death, but also in all of these cases people may be unable to cope with the consequences of their illness. However, given that little can be done medically, it is one's moral interests that most people would be concerned with; that is, in those cases where medicine has little or nothing to offer, one would be more interested in ensuring that one's moral beliefs and values took precedence over futile medical care. Finally, as we noted earlier, only 11.5% of the population is hospitalized each year and 15% of those hospitalized consume some 55% of hospital expenditures (Gagner 1992, p. 26).[75]

If we sum the percentages of office visits that can be safely handled by non-physician practitioners, 80% of adult visits and 90% of pediatric office visits, with the percentage of people hospitalized each year, the result would be almost 100%. If we assume that, roughly, half of the people hospitalized each year are adults and the other half are children, then that covers, respectively 85.75% of adults and 95.75% of children. Given that the leading causes of death are such that there is little that physicians can do with respect to curing the condition, then there remains only a small percentage of the population each year who are afflicted as the asymmetry of information problem presupposes. In addition, the justification for applying the principle of weak paternalism is also weakened, for contrary to what most people may have thought, there is only a small percentage of people who need to be protected from harming themselves due to an inability to understand the complexity of modern medicine.

While Arrow's attempted justification of the medical profession's non-market system of medical services is a possible solution to the problem of market failure, it is not the only solution and neither should it be the most preferred solution. In earlier chapters, we outlined some of the many deficiencies of the meta-structure of health care. We identified the problem of higher costs due to physicians inducing demand for their services, not to mention the costs consumers suffer in terms of increased risks for injuries as a result of this unnecessary and inappropriate medical care and their consequent lack of consenting to these procedures. In addition to the unnecessary and inappropriate care resulting from physicians inducing demand for their services, there was the more general problem of physicians providing unnecessary medical care. We also identified the problems of fraud, self-referral and physician ownership of medical diagnostic and therapeutic centers and equipment. All of these practices are in violation of Gauthier's proviso, for they better the provider of health care at the expense of the consumer of health care. This conclusion is augmented by the fact that only a small percentage of the population are responsible for consuming the vast majority of health care expenditures, that the institution of medicine, as opposed to the individual practitioner of medicine, has been "irrelevant in the determination of aggregate social indices whatever comfort it may have brought to particular individuals" (Hartwell 1974, p. 3), and that 80% of basic adult care and 90% of pediatric care could safely be delegated to non-physician practitioners of health care.

Furthermore, the medical profession in both Canada and the United States has received enormous public subsidies in terms of public funding of hospitals, medical schools, and research. For example, in the United States federal and state funding for construction of medical facilities in 1929 was $213 million (Gibson 1979, p. 23) and it has steadily increased since then. In 1990 in the United States expenditures for construction of medical facilities amounted to $10.4 billion (Levit *et al*, 1991b, p. 47) and it is projected to increase to $17.5 billion by the year 2000 (Sonnefeld *et al*, 1991, p. 17). Federal and state funding of medical research, which amounted to only $3 million in 1940 (Gibson 1979, p. 23), climbed to $12.4 billion in 1990 (Levit *et al*, 1991b, p. 47), and is projected to increase to $22.3 billion by the turn of the century (Sonnefeld *et al*, 1991, p. 17).

The figures given above are representative of what is spent annually on both research and construction of medical facilities by both the federal and state governments. The situation in

Canada differs only in the amount spent. Not only does this mean that the medical profession does not have to bear all the costs associated with the accumulation of knowledge needed to practice their profession, they also do not need to bear all the costs for the tools they need to practice their profession, nor even the buildings they need to practice in. Furthermore, the medical profession, through officially sanctioned organizations, actively seeks voluntary donations in terms of charitable contributions and the donation of particular organs and entire bodies. These contributions allow members of the medical profession to further their knowledge base at little or no cost to themselves. However, given that these contributions are voluntary, there is no violation of Gauthier's proviso.

The consumer's position, on the other hand, has been worsened by the action of the medical profession and in several respects: people would have greater access to medical care and the price of medical care would be lower if there were more physicians, price discrimination was not in effect, and there was no institutional ban on competitive advertising. Individuals could seek out non-physician practitioners for the treatment of minor illnesses; this would not only lower the cost of medical services by increasing the supply of people who could provide treatments, it would also give people greater access to those services. People who could not afford the price of a physician, or those who did not want to go to a physician for services that non-physician practitioners of health care could perform just as well, would have alternatives available to them.

Not only does the consumer suffer from the disadvantage of being unable to seek cheaper forms of treatment by going to non-physician practitioners of health care, she is also prohibited from treating herself for even minor bacteriological infections and pains from non-life threatening injuries. For example, it does not take a decade of higher education to diagnose most bacteriological infections, nor is such knowledge required to treat such infections. The procedure for diagnosing and treating such conditions is now so standardized that it is easily imparted to first year nursing students. One need only take a culture from the infected site and then send the culture to a laboratory for a sensitivity test (a simple test performed by a laboratory technician which determines what drug would best treat a given bacteria). Armed with such knowledge, one need only obtain the drug and take it for the recommended number of days. The number of days recommended may vary, depending on the drug, the bacteria, and the site of the infection but this is hardly an impediment to the non-physician practitioner for successfully treating either herself or another. Nor is it an insurmountable obstacle to treating one's self, for the information is easily available to anyone at the price of looking it up in a book or extracting it from one's own personal computer (Ferguson 1992).

Moreover, not only does it not require medical expertise to do these simple procedures, which is evidenced by the simple fact that physicians employ nurses to do these and various other procedures, it does not require medical expertise to know that one is in pain after having broken a limb and that an analgesic will relieve the discomfort. Most broken limbs, for example, are not only set by technicians but the cast is also applied by technicians. The only reason why one must see a physician when one has a broken limb is that the medical profession has sole dominion over prescribing the drugs necessary to relieve the accompanying pain.

We raise the issues of lesser trained professionals and self-treatment not just because the compulsory prohibition of them is in violation of Gauthier's proviso, but also to make another simpler point. That point is that a great many of the practices and procedures which currently fall under the domain of medicine (which, we remind the reader, is defined by the medical profession itself) not only need not fall under the domain of medicine, but they could also be performed by anyone who took the time and trouble to acquire some simple basic knowledge. The cost of medical care is high and, as we have argued, it is higher than what it might be under a free market system. If we are concerned with reducing the cost of medical care as well as providing increased access to health care, then we would be well advised to encourage people to acquire and use the basic knowledge and skills necessary to treat themselves for the many minor ills and injuries that threaten us frequently throughout our lives.

While there might be paternalistic arguments that could be made to prevent people who did not have the requisite knowledge and skills from treating themselves, there should be no principled objection to allowing people who demonstrated competence with respect to the requisite knowledge and skills to treat themselves. In addition, for those who demonstrated sufficient competence their should be no principled objection to their diagnosing and/or treating others who came to them for such assistance. The competency of these would-be non-physician practitioners could be ascertained in a number of ways. For example, as Arrow correctly notes, certification of competency could accomplish the same goals as the current practice of medical licensure. Not only would this increase the supply of health-care providers, thus resulting in greater access for more people at lower costs, but it would also make more efficient use of a physician's time and his expertise. Furthermore, such an approach would still leave open the option of seeking out medical advice should one wish to do so.

If one were to consider what rational agents, under Gauthier's theory of justice, might agree to with respect to the issue of justice between the provider of health care services and the consumer of health care services, given the noted deficiencies of the present meta-structure of health care, as well as the benefits individual clinicians provide to individual patients, the results would be different than the existing systems in both Canada and the United States. As a possible bargain the existing system of health care delivery in both Canada and the United States is surely one rational consumers of health care would reject, and for several reasons.

Let us begin by first considering the reasons why rational consumers of health care would not agree to a bargain that implemented a Canadian-style system of health care delivery. Rational consumers of health care would not agree to a bargain that implemented a Canadian system of health care delivery for it benefits mainly the poor and that small minority that consumes the vast majority of a country's health care budget. That is, they would object to the compulsory redistribution of wealth that takes place in order to ensure that everyone has access to medical care. Rational consumers of health care would object to this compulsory redistribution of wealth on the grounds that it violates Gauthier's proviso, for it makes some better off by worsening the situation of others. The second reason why rational consumers of health care would not agree to a bargain that implemented a Canadian-style system of health care delivery is that they would object to the medical profession's monopoly on the practice of medicine. Not only is the medical profession's monopoly of the practice of medicine in violation of Gauthier's proviso, it also prohibits an individual from exercising her liberty to care for her own health and/or seeking out other non-physician practitioners to assist her in meeting her health care needs, wants, and/or desires.

One might want to object that Gauthier's rational bargainers would be ignorant of their future health care needs and therefore they would not reason as we have argued above. We grant that such bargainers would indeed be ignorant of their future health care needs, but from this it does not follow that they would not reason as we argued. On the contrary, they would reason as we suggest, for while they would be ignorant of their particular future health care needs, they would know that they would have future health care needs; that is, while they would be ignorant of their particular future health care needs, they would not be ignorant concerning their need for health care in the future. Nor would they be ignorant of the empirical data we have presented throughout the course of our investigation. They would have knowledge of the existing deficiencies in the present non-market system of medical services. They would know, for example, that physicians have been unable to sufficiently constrain their economic interests such that they could refrain from inducing demand for medical care. They would have knowledge of the problem of both nosocomial infections and iatrogenic injuries. They would be aware of the problems of medical fraud and physician self-referral. In addition, they would be aware of the contribution that non-medical practitioners of health care could make if not prohibited from doing so, of the fact that 90% of patient contacts with the health care system are for the management of chronic conditions, and the small percentages of people who would be seriously ill. Given this knowledge, even though they are ignorant of their own particular future health care needs, rational bargainers would reason as I suggested above.

If we now consider whether rational consumers of health care would agree to a bargain that implemented an American-style system of health care delivery, we will find that they would object to such a system for the same reasons they objected to the Canadian-style system of health care delivery. They would object to the American medical profession's monopoly on the practice of medicine and they would object to the compulsory redistribution of wealth that the American system of health care delivery rests on. In addition, they would object to an American-style system of health care delivery, for not only does it preclude an individual from exercising her liberty to meet her own health care needs and wants and/or employing non-physician practitioners to assist her in this endeavor, but the American system of health care delivery has precluded some 37 million Americans from having access to health care insurance. The only potential benefit in such a bargain for roughly 90% of health care consumers is that if they are unable to pay for the health care services they need, then it is possible that they might receive the health care services they need regardless of their ability to pay.

However, such assurances are of little or no comfort, when, finding himself unable to pay for his health care needs, a person is not only denied health care but also precluded from either acting on his own to secure his own health or seeking out non-physician practitioners of health care who might be able to assist him in meeting his health care needs. Moreover, assurances are not guarantees and if the consumer of health care has no guarantee that he will receive the health care he needs when he needs it, then it would not be individually rational for him to agree to such an arrangement, or so we shall argue.

Individual rationality is defined in terms of maximizing one's expected utility. An outcome is not Pareto optimal when some person can be made better off without making any other person worse off. Thus, for example, to say on behalf of an American health care consumer that agreeing to an American-style system of health care delivery would not be individually rational is to say that for that consumer of health care, she is worse off under the existing system of health care delivery than she would be under an alternative system of health care delivery. If we assume that having the option of either seeking alternative less-qualified people to diagnose and treat one's self in the event of illness and/or injury, or the option of diagnosing and treating one's self, is preferable to having no option in the event of being unable to get medical care because one cannot pay for it, or it is unavailable where one lives, then one is worse off than what one would be under a system of health care delivery that provided her with these options. The existing system of health care delivery would be individually rational for a given individual if it made her no worse off than an alternative system of health care delivery. Under this alternative system of health care delivery, an individual would be free to either care for her own health to the best of her ability or to seek out whomsoever she chose to assist her in meeting her health care needs. Under the existing system of health care delivery in the United States neither of these options are available to her. Moreover, she is not guaranteed that she will have the requisite access to meet her health care needs should she be unable to pay. Therefore the existing system of health care delivery is not individually rational for her. Generalizing this conclusion we can say that the existing system of health care delivery is not individually rational for all individuals who are in the position such that they would be better off under an alternative system of health care delivery. In the United States, this amounts to a significant number of people, some 37 million.

The argument above assumes, of course, that having more options never makes one worse off. While this is a common assumption in economics and rational choice theory, it may not always be warranted (Dworkin 1982; Titmuss 1971; Arrow 1981; Singer 1981). But given not only the uncertainty associated with the incidence of disease and the uncertainty associated with the efficacy of treatment, but also the uncertainty of being able to receive treatment in the event of illness and inability to pay, having the option of diagnosing and treating one's self or the option of seeking out non-physician practitioners of health care to diagnose and treat one's self in the event of illness is certainly preferable when one could be (or is) denied access to health care services because of the inability to pay.

The existing systems of health care in both Canada and the United States are unjust, or so we have argued, for they are in violation of Gauthier's proviso. If Gauthier's proviso is violated, then those whose rights were violated, or whose liberties were unjustifiably restricted, are owed market compensation. Health care consumers in both Canada and the United States have had their liberty unjustifiably restricted with respect to either caring for their own health or using non-physician practitioners of health care. They are, therefore, owed market compensation. The amount of compensation health care consumers are owed is a just minimum of health care and health care consumers are morally entitled to it. This conclusion, of course, presupposes that, as we have argued pace Arrow, the medical profession's monopoly on the practice of medicine is indeed unjustified.

Let us now assume, for the sake of argument, that the medical profession's monopoly on the practice of medicine is justified. If the medical profession's monopoly on the practice of medicine is indeed justified -- that is, giving the medical profession a monopoly on the practice of medicine does not violate the Pareto optimality condition -- then it would follow that restricting a person's liberty would not require compensation. And if compensation were not owed, then, someone might argue, according to our argument, people would not be entitled to a just minimum of health care. However, just because people are not owed compensation for justified restrictions of their liberty, it does not follow that they are not entitled to a just minimum of health care. For being entitled to a just minimum of health care does not just rest upon the moral claim of being owed compensation for the unjustified restriction of one's liberty. A moral claim for a just minimum of health care can also be found in securing for each person their fair share of the cooperative benefits of allowing the medical profession a monopoly on the practice of medicine.

If we assume, as we did above, that the medical profession's monopoly on the practice of medicine is indeed justified, then, in order for the Pareto optimality condition to be satisfied, it must be the case that giving the medical profession a monopoly on the practice of medicine allows us to obtain benefits which would otherwise be unobtainable. That is to say we are better off in a situation where the medical profession has a monopoly than in a situation where the medical profession does not have a monopoly. Or, to put it another way, there are more benefits to be obtained if the medical profession has a monopoly than if the medical profession does not have a monopoly. However, if there are more benefits obtained by allowing the medical profession to have a monopoly than not allowing the monopoly, then, since every person contributes to the production of these benefits by the (assumed) justified restriction of their liberty, while they are not owed compensation, they are entitled to their fair share of these benefits as determined by Gauthier's principle of distributive justice, minimax relative concession. Since each person's liberty has been restricted so that the benefits can be obtained, each is entitled, as determined by minimax relative concession, to their fair share of the benefits realized. The share that each person would be entitled to if the restriction of their liberty was a justified restriction of liberty -- and by assumption it is -- is a just minimum of health care.

In summary our main argument for a just minimum of health care is a disjunctive syllogism. Either it is the case that the medical profession's monopoly on the practice of medicine, a non-market solution to the problem of market failure, is justified or it is not. Arrow argued that the non-market solution was justified; we argued it was not. If Arrow is correct and the restriction of people's liberty is indeed justified, then according to Gauthier's principle of distributive justice, minimax relative concession, each is entitled to their fair share of the benefits obtained by restricting people's liberty and giving the medical profession a monopoly on the practice of medicine. If we are correct and the restrictions on people's liberty are not justified, then people are owed market compensation for the unjustified restriction of their liberty. In either case, people have a positive right to a just minimum of health care; that is, they are either entitled to their fair share of the benefits of allowing the medical profession a monopoly on the practice of medicine or they are entitled to compensation for the unjustified restriction of their liberty which results from the medical profession having a monopoly on the practice of medicine.

Given the injustice of both the Canadian and American systems of health care delivery outlined above, two options suggest themselves. On the one hand we could attempt to model a possible bargain between providers and consumers of health care, taking care to ensure that the condition of individual rationality was satisfied and that Gauthier's proviso was not violated. On the other hand, we could attempt to modify the existing system in such a way as to remove the injustices. While we cannot here go into any detail with respect to each of these two alternatives, we can suggest what such a system of just health care delivery might amount to.

Regardless of which of the two options was chosen we should expect that people have, if not the liberty to care for their own health either by self-diagnosis and treatment or by seeking out non-physician practitioners of health care to do this for them, then the equivalent of this. That people have either the liberty to care for their own health or some equivalent thereof should not be underestimated in terms of its value. For, regardless of the form such an equivalent might take, while it might not be a "decent minimum" of health care it will be a just minimum of health care and people will have a positive right to it.

Lest we compound the existing injustice by continuing with a course of action which is not morally justified, we as a society should at least pause to consider how we might proceed from where we currently are. In the following chapter we shall attempt to outline some of the main implications of our argument for a just minimum of health care. In particular, we shall focus on how our conclusion that people are entitled to a just minimum of health care could affect the existing systems of health care delivery in both Canada and the United States. We shall argue that there are three possible interpretations of the just minimum of health care and that Gauthier's principle of minimax relative concession can be employed, at least in theory, to determine what the just minimum of health care might amount to. In addition, we shall also show how our argument for a just minimum of health care avoids the difficulties faced by both Daniels' fair equality of opportunity argument for health care and Buchanan's enforced beneficence argument for a decent minimum of health care.

Chapter VII
From Theory to Practice

A society operating in accord with Gauthier's principles of justice is, to use Gauthier's term, an "essentially just society" (Gauthier 1986, p. 341). And while an essentially just society can neither ban nor require a free market in health care, it must remove barriers to a free market in health care; that is, it must remove the unjustified restrictions on people's liberty to meet their own health care needs, wants, and/or desires, lest it remain in violation of Gauthier's proviso. Should society choose to retain a non-market system of health care delivery, then, as it will be in violation of Gauthier's proviso, citizens of that society will have a positive right to the just minimum of health care. We shall not here attempt to adjudicate which of these alternatives, the free market or the non-market system of health care delivery, is the preferred alternative, for our task in this chapter is to provide further support for our argument for the concept of the just minimum of health care by showing how it avoids the difficulties to which both Daniels' and Buchanan's arguments succumbed. In concluding this chapter, we shall attempt to show how Gauthier's principle of minimax relative concession can be used to determine, at least in principle, what people are entitled to with respect to the just minimum of health care and how the implementation of a just minimum of health care would affect the non-market systems of health care delivery in Canada and the United States.

Under Gauthier's theory of justice people do have a positive right to a just minimum of health care; that is, people are entitled to exercise their liberty with respect to meeting their own health care needs, wants, and/or desires or they are entitled to market compensation for the unjustified restrictions on the exercise of their liberty to meet those needs, wants, and/or desires. In either case, it is just, it is a minimum, and people have a positive right to it. And people can use their entitlement to the just minimum of health care to meet their health care needs, their health care wants, and/or their health care desires, at least insofar as their limited resources allow.

One should not interpret the just minimum to mean that this is the maximum amount of health care people may be entitled to consume, for this is not the case. People may be entitled to more than the just minimum if they can pay the market price for that which they wish to obtain over and above the just minimum. Of course, not all people who need, want, and/or desire more than the just minimum may have the resources to obtain more than the just minimum. If they do not have the resources to obtain what they need, want, and/or desire in excess of the just minimum and no one is voluntarily willing to provide them with those resources, then, as a strict matter of justice, while this may be unfortunate, it is not unjust (Engelhardt 1981, pp. 121-137). Using Gauthier's terms we can say that the just minimum of health care does not violate Gauthier's proviso; by denying a person more health care than what they are entitled to -- that is, more than the just minimum -- we are merely failing to better their situation and not worsening their situation and therefore Gauthier's proviso is not violated.

There is a limit to what justice requires and under Gauthier's theory of justice the just minimum of health care is, we have argued, all that justice requires. People are, however, beneficent. We documented the evidence of this beneficence -- at least American beneficence -- in Chapter IV, where we argued that American's may have met their duty of beneficence. Recall that American's contributed, voluntarily, almost $104 billion to charitable causes in 1988. The total voluntarily contributed amount, although it was not all donated to health care related concerns, was roughly equal to 19% of the $546 billion spent on health care in the United States in 1988. The amount contributed to health care related concerns, roughly $20 billion, exceeded the Government Accounting Office's estimate that it would need $18 billion to insure those American's without health care insurance. If American's continued voluntarily to contribute to charity, then the amount contributed could be used to assist those who needed more health care than what they were entitled to as a strict matter of justice. With the additional assistance that charity provided, people would be better situated to meet their health care needs, wants, and/or desires.

In addition to providing everyone with a just minimum of health care and allowing them to use their entitlement to the just minimum of health care to meet at least some of their health care needs, wants, and/or desires, the just minimum of health care also solves the theory-dependent version of the bottomless pit problem. The theory-dependent version of the bottomless pit problem is resolved for the just minimum of health care limits the amount of health care resources that everyone is justly entitled to receive. Everyone is equally entitled to receive the just minimum of health care, plus whatever amount they can obtain in excess of the just minimum either by spending their own resources or through the voluntary contributions of others. In Chapter III we argued that there were three considerations of the theory-dependent version of the bottomless pit problem that made it deeply problematic: the morbidity, the supply, and the cost/benefit problems. The just minimum of health care renders each of these considerations otiose, for the just minimum of health care directly constrains the consumption of health care resources.

Regardless of how sick and/or injured people are, they are only entitled to the just minimum of health care. If a person's health care needs exceeds what they are entitled to *via* the just minimum, then they are not entitled to what they need. The just minimum of health care does not guarantee that everyone will receive the amount of health care they need, but rather only the just minimum of health care. If the cost of treating someone's medical condition is less than the amount remaining on that person's account, then that person could choose to undergo the treatment and have the cost deducted from his account. If the cost of treating the condition exceeded the balance of his account, and he had additional insurance, then that additional insurance could be used to pay the excess amount. If he had no additional insurance, then he could access the charitable funds that were available. If the charitable funds available were suffi-cient to meet the costs of his treatment, then those funds could be used to supplement his entitlement to the just minimum. We can imagine -- given that charity, like justice, also has its limits -- the person in question had, for example, previously consumed his charitable amount. If this was the case, then, unfortunately but not unjustly, he would not be entitled to receive the treatment. While this may offend some people's moral sensibilities, it is not unjust. We live in a world of limited resources and while this is also unfortunate, it too is not unjust. In the above example the cost of treating the person exceeded the just minimum of health care and what he might have obtained through charity and/or his own resources. Therefore, on our account, he has, as a strict matter of justice, no further claims to health care.

The just minimum of health care also renders the supply problem less intractable, for the just minimum specifies a limit to what people are entitled to receive. If people are limited to what they can receive, then -- since what people can maximally receive as a strict matter of justice is limited to the just minimum -- the number of people who can receive the just minimum will be greatly enhanced. In theory, however, there is no limit to the number of people who can receive the just minimum of health care. For, since everyone is entitled to exercise their liberty with respect to meeting their own health care needs, or market com-pensation for the unjustified restriction of their liberty, or their fair share of the benefits of the medical profession having a monopoly on the practice of medicine as determined by minimax relative concession then, while additional people could render the minimum amount less than what it might be if there were less people, it would not alter the content of the just minimum.

In addition to resolving the morbidity and the supply prob-lems the just minimum of health care also resolves the cost/bene-fit problem. In order to see how the just minimum resolves this latter problem, let us consider how the just minimum of health care might be actualized in the real world. Imagine, for example, that the just minimum amounted to $100,000 of health care over the course of a person's lifetime. Imagine further that every citizen was given a credit card with this $100,000 credited to their account. In addition to containing the credited amount, the card might also contain a patient's complete medical history and any other medical related data, such as allergies, *et cetera*. The patient could simply present her card to her non-physician practitioner or her physician -- the choice would be hers -- and the health care practitioner would have instant access not only to her medical data but also her total remaining balance. Since each person would be entitled to the just minimum of health care, each person would decide whether to use her just minimum for particular treatments or for early detection and prevention. If, for example, a patient chose to have a guaiac test to determine if she had colorectal cancer, then the amount of that test would be deducted from her account. Since her health care resources would be limited, she would be prudent to carefully choose how she would consume those resources. If she chose to consume her health care resources in such a way that the cost exceeded the benefits, then she would quickly reach the limit that the just minimum of health care guaranteed and she would be not be entitled to any further health care, unless she had her own resources or could draw from charitable sources. Thus by ensuring that everyone is entitled to the just minimum of health care, we ensure that either they will consume those resources wisely or they will quickly consume their just minimum. Regardless of which of the above two alternatives is endorsed by society, the amount that each person can consume is limited by the just minimum and the amount that each person does consume is a reflection of their preferences. If some people prefer, given that they have a limited health care budget, early detection and prevention then they will be able to satisfy their preferences. If other people do not share their preferences, then they will make alternative decisions about how they want to consume their limited health care budget. In either case, since the amount of health care each person can consume is limited, then the total amount of health care that people can consume is also limited and the cost/benefit problem is also resolved.

The just minimum of health care ensures that people will either be responsible with respect to consuming their limited health care budget or be prevented from free-riding on their other more health conscious neighbors. Thus the just minimum of health care, like Daniels' theory of justice in health care, does not "deny individuals the autonomy to take risks that endanger life, liver, and lungs" (Daniels 1985, p. 153). However, unlike Daniels' theory of justice in health care, the just minimum of health care does ensure that people will be responsible for their actions when it does come to endangering life, liver, and lungs. It ensures that people will be responsible by limiting the amount of health care resources that they can consume. If some people have resources over and above the just minimum of health care, then they can engage in the aforementioned behaviors but their doing so will not enable them to evade their personal responsibilities when it comes to paying the medical cost associated with engaging in such activities.

Unlike Buchanan's notion of a decent minimum, the concept of a just minimum is conceptually connected to health care. On the one hand, the just minimum is conceptually connected to health care for the just minimum is what health care people would be entitled to if their liberty to meet their own health care needs was not unjustifiably restricted. On the other hand, if we view the just minimum in terms of receiving market compensation for the unjustified restriction of people's liberty to meet their own health care needs, then the conceptual connection is that the just minimum is payment in kind -- that is, health care -- for the unjustified restriction of people's liberty to meet their own health care needs. And finally, if we view the just minimum in terms of people's fair share of the benefits obtained from the medical profession's monopoly on the practice of medicine, then, as above, the conceptual connection is that the just minimum is payment in kind for the benefits which they are owed.

The just minimum of health care, we have argued, overcomes the difficulties identified in both Daniels' and Buchanan's arguments. We now want to identify both how Gauthier's principle of minimax relative concession can be used to determine, at least in theory, what the just minimum would amount to in practice and the main implication of our argument for the just minimum of health care for the non-market systems of health care delivery in both Canada and the United States.

There is a difficulty in using Gauthier's principle of minimax relative concession to determine what the just minimum of health care would amount to in practice. For in order to determine what the just minimum of health care would amount to in practice presupposes that we can determine what the baseline of medical knowledge and care would have been in the absence of the unjustified restrictions of people's liberties. The difficulty in determining the baseline is twofold: first, we have no means for determining how far back we ought to go to find the baseline;

and second, which of the several possible baselines is the baseline that ought to be used to determine the point from which compensation is to be paid. We will not attempt to resolve these theoretical problems here, for any such attempt would take us far beyond the scope of our original inquiry. However, we can imagine that there is a unique baseline that can be determined and proceed with our investigations under this assumption.

Gauthier's principle of minimax relative concession, he argues, is the principle that rational agents would agree on to govern the distribution of the cooperative surplus. The cooperative surplus, given the limited context of our investigation, is the difference in social/medical benefits between what would have been obtained in a free market for health care and what social/medical benefits have actually been obtained by a society that has unjustifiably restricted the liberty of its citizens to meet their own health care needs, wants, and/or desires. We assume that there is such a difference, for if there was no difference (or if the difference was a negative value), then whatever justification there might have been for a non-market system of health care delivery could be shown to be demonstrably false.

As we saw in Chapter V, if contributions to the cooperative surplus are relatively equal, then each party to the agreement would agree to the distribution that minimized the maximum concession any person had to make. If each party contributed an equal amount to the cooperative enterprise, then their concessions should also be equal such that each party to the agreement ought to receive an equal share of the benefits. The share of the benefits that each person ought to receive would be the just minimum of health care. If we assume, counterfactually, that each party did not contribute equally to the cooperative enterprise, then the share of the benefits that each person would be entitled to would be proportional to their contribution. We claim that this latter assumption is a counterfactual assumption for the reason that each party as a private citizen, in terms of the unjustified restriction of their liberty, did indeed equally contribute to the cooperative enterprise. However, one might want to argue that physicians, since they had a monopoly on the practice of medicine and therefore did not suffer from a comparable restriction of liberty, did not make the same contribution as other citizens.

This objection fails to note that the agreement under consideration is a hypothetical agreement, not an actual agreement, and that physicians would only have their monopoly *ex post*. That is, the parties to this hypothetical agreement make their agreement not on the premise of real world considerations, but rather hypothetical considerations. In other words, the question under consideration is not "what would we agree to given that physicians have a monopoly on the practice of medicine?" Rather, the question is "what would we agree to if physicians were to have a monopoly on the practice of medicine and our liberty to meet our health care needs, wants, and/or desires was thereby restricted?" In the former case, as we have argued, they would agree to market compensation for the unjustified restrictions on their liberty. This, we argued, was equivalent to what they could have obtained in the absence of the unjustified restrictions on their liberty. We are now attempting to ascertain what they would agree to *ex ante* not *ex post*; that is, we are now attempting to ascertain what they would agree to with respect to the division of the cooperative surplus obtained from giving the medical profession a monopoly on the practice of medicine. In this case, as we argued when we assumed that the restriction of one's liberty was indeed justified, they would agree to an equal distribution since their contribution to the cooperative enterprise, in terms of the restrictions on their liberty, would be equal.

We have argued that people are morally entitled to a just minimum of health care. We now want to briefly explicate the main implication of our argument for the distribution of health care in both Canada and the United States. As we noted earlier we will not attempt here to adjudicate whether Canada and/or the United States ought to adopt a free market in health care or a non-market system of health care. As a simplifying assumption we shall assume that both countries will continue with their non-market systems of health care. Given this assumption, our final task is to ascertain the main implication of our argument for a just minimum of health care to the existing non-market systems of health care in both countries. We shall begin with Canada and conclude with the United States.

The main implication of our argument for the just minimum of health care in Canada is that people would no longer be entitled to as much health care as they are now legally entitled to receive. For in Canada the amount of health care Canadians are legally entitled to receive is greater than what they would be entitled to receive under our argument for the just minimum of health care, at least we assume this to be the case. If this assumption proved to be false, a question we shall not attempt to answer, then they would be entitled to more health care but the amount they would be entitled to receive could not exceed what they would be entitled to under the just minimum of health care. The second main implication of our argument for the just minimum of health care -- that is if Canadians were entitled to less than what they are now legally entitled to receive -- is that Canadians would have to devise social support systems such that those whose medical needs could not be met under the just minimum of health care would have some assistance in coping with the new moral order in health care.

The main implication of our argument for the just minimum of health care in the United States is that those who currently have no access to health care, typically the uninsured and perhaps even the under-insured, would have to be given access to health care. That is, those who currently receive less than what they are entitled to receive by virtue of the just minimum of health care would be entitled to what the just minimum requires, lest Gauthier's proviso continues to be violated. Those who are receiving more than they are justly entitled to receive by virtue of the just minimum -- that is, those who are not supplementing the just minimum with their own resources or charitable resources -- would have their existing entitlement curtailed. If this latter condition obtained, then the United States, like Canada, should devise social support systems that would assist these people to deal with the new moral order in health care.

These are the main implications of our argument for the just minimum of health care. There are, of course, other implications of our argument for both countries but we shall not identify them here. Nor shall we attempt to explicate how either Canada or the United States could (or ought to) implement the just minimum of health care. We leave both of these tasks for a future occasion, for we have accomplished what we set out to do; that is, we have established that people do have a moral positive right to a just minimum of health care. Some may find the just minimum of health care to be inadequate; others may find it excessive. We, however, find it to be just and people are morally entitled to it.

Notes

1 Another important element in the deprofessionalization of medicine is the "deskilling" or "routinization" of medical procedures (Light and Levine, 1988, p. 15; Stoeckle 1988, p. 81).

2 The terms are sometimes used interchangeably to characterize the fall from grace that the institution of medicine is currently undergoing. There are, of course, difficulties with definitions for both concepts and work is underway to clarify exactly what these terms might mean. *Cf* Friedson (1986), chap. 2 and Hafferty (1988), pp. 202-225.

3 An adverse event is defined as "injuries resulting from medical intervention" (Hiatt *et al*, 1989, p. 480). One should note that the Harvard study was published in three parts, not including an initial overview and two follow-up articles by authors involved in the original study. Hence, for reference purposes, see the following in the following order: Hiatt *et al*, 1989; Brennan *et al*, February 7, 1991; Leape *et al*, February 7, 1991; Localio *et al*, 1991; and Weiler *et al*, 1992.

4 Also see Brahams (1989).

5 George Lundberg, editor of *JAMA*, the journal which published this study, as well as the article by Crane which is referred to below, is reported to have said with respect to the validity of the results of these two studies, that "we believe they [the results of the study] are all valid as they stand" (McCormick 1992, p. 92).

6 The authors of this study also state that these figures actually "understate the proportion of physicians involved in direct patient care who participate in joint venture arrangements" (Mitchell and Scott, 1992, p. 84), and for two reasons. First,

not all facilities responded to the requests for ownership information. Furthermore, as the authors also indicated, follow-up phone calls revealed that the facilities that did not respond were more likely to be involved in such joint ventures. Second, the study did not include all types of health care facilities such as centers which provide medical services for lithotripsy, home infusion therapy, kidney dialysis, weight loss, substance abuse, pharmacies, and orthotic and prosthetic devices.

7   The profits from self-referring physicians can be enormous. One doctor is reported to have secured a 420% return on his investment (Morgenson 1991, p. 38).

8   For an account of how Gauthier's theory might be applied to the issue of informed consent, see my "Hypothetical Contractarianism and the Disclosure Requirement Problem in Informed Consent" (1991).

9   The AMA Council on Ethical and Judicial Affairs has recently endorsed the practice of physician self-referrals, notwithstanding their profession ethic against such practices. In fact, Daniel Johnson, speaker of the AMA House of Delegates, in commenting on the issue of self-referral, said "it is not unprecedented for delegates to adopt policy inconsistent with AMA ethical opinions" (McCormick 1992, p. 1). In 1986 the AMA Council, in order to "prevent abuses of self-referral," issued "safeguards." In 1989 these "safeguards" (AMA Council on Ethical and Judicial Affairs, 1992, p. 2366) were upgraded to "guidelines." In 1992, in response to the empirical evidence presented above, the AMA "endorsed the often-criticized practice of doctors sending patients for tests at labs in which those physicians have a financial interest" (Burton 1992, p. B12). The AMA's rationale for endorsing this much maligned practice rested on a "distinction between the physician who benefits financially from services that the physician actually provides and the physician who benefits purely from the ability to refer patients for services" (AMA Council on Ethical and Judicial Affairs, 1992, p. 2368).

10   Another problem concerning laboratories is the increasing number of doctors who have labs in their offices. One American study found that there was anywhere from 50% to

250% (Crawley *et al*, 1986, p. 374) variability in the lab results of doctors who had labs in their offices and independently owned licensed laboratories. The reasons for this are several, but of particular note is the high turnover rate of personnel in doctor's labs and the fact that many "had little or no post-high school education" (Crawley *et al*, 1986, p. 376). It was studies such as this which led the American federal government, *via* the Clinical Laboratory Improvement Amendments of 1988, to place "all physician office laboratories under government scrutiny" (Eastman 1992, p. 13).

11 Procedure-coding creep occurs when a physician selects a code, when billing Medicare, that has a higher level of reimbursement than alternative codes. For example, when billing for office visits the physician can choose one of four codes: brief, limited, intermediate, or extended. The amount of reimbursement is tied to the code chosen, with brief having the lowest amount attached to it and extended having the highest amount of reimbursement attached to it. For an account of this phenomenon in Canada see Barer and Evans (1992), pp. 13-15.

12 Prior to presenting the evidence supporting the view that physicians induce demand for their services, we note in passing that 82.6% of health economists agree that physicians do indeed induce demand for their services (Feldman and Morrisey, 1990, p. 641).

13 The theoretical literature on the problem of induced demand is extensive but for an overview of some of the conceptual problems see Green (1987) pp. 21-34; Stano (1985) pp. 197-211 and (1987) pp. 227-238; Farley (1986) pp. 315-333; Feldman (1988) pp. 239-261; Rice and Labelle (1989) pp. 587-600; and Feldman and Sloan's reply to the Rice and Labelle article (1989) pp. 621-625; Cromwell and Mitchell (1986) pp. 293-313; Reinhardt (1985) pp. 187-193; Rice (1987) pp. 375-376; Wedig *et al* (1989) pp. 601-620; and McGuire and Pauly (1991) pp. 385-410.

14 A study of dental services in Norway concluded "that demand and utilization of dental services in the Norwegian adult population increases when population:dentist ratio decreases *ceterus paribus*," and that "a reduction in the preva-

lence of dental diseases may not necessarily lead to a concurrent reduction in demand and utilization of dental services" (Grytten *et al*, 1990, p. 490). Another study of dentists, in the United Kingdom, found that "considerable support is found for the inducement hypothesis" and that "the results imply that in areas of abundant supplies of dentists, incomes are enhanced by the provision of services in excess of what is required" (Birch 1988, p. 146).

15 For a more detailed account of how provinces in Canada have attempted to control fees, see Lomas *et al*, (1989), "Paying Physicians in Canada: Minding Our P's and Q's." The reference to minding their P's and Q's in the title of this article was put in because it "underlines the care that had to be taken by the provinces when dealing with the medical profession" (Lomas *et al*, 1989, p. 95) on the issue of fees. For more details on Quebec in particular, see Contandriopoulos (1986).

16 Lomas *et al*, note that if physicians cannot increase utilization of physician services because of the expenditure caps on their fees, then they switch to using "more costly types of services" (Lomas *et al*, 1989, p. 94).

17 For further details on British Columbia attempt to legislate on restricting the supply of physicians see Barer (1988).

18 This study updates and augments Barer *et al* previous study. For Barer's response see Barer (1991).

19 In fact, Fuchs and Hahn found that "physician fees for procedures are 234 percent higher in the United States than in Canada" (Fuchs and Hahn, 1990, p. 886).

20 Also see Crichton *et al*, 1990, p. 218; Coburn 1988, p. 104.

21 Another poll, conducted on behalf of the American Medical Association (AMA), indicated that "nearly three-quarters of Americans believe the cost of medical care, insurance or drugs is the main problem facing the U.S. healthcare system" (Anderson 1992, p. 7). In another poll, conducted in January 1992, respondents ranked health care and health insurance highest among their concerns. With respect to a future presidential State of the Union Address, a very substantial majority of Americans, 93%, wanted it to include a program for health care reform (Blendon *et al*, 1992, p. 2509). Earlier

studies (Gabel *et al*, 1989, pp. 103-118; Jajich-Toth and Roper, 1990, pp. 149-157) however, reveal that there may be some inconsistencies and contradictions in American's views on the importance of health care.

22   From 1985 to 1990 "the average annual cost of a worker's medical bills and insurance -- what both employees and employers pay -- nearly doubled. The A. Foster Higgins consulting firm projects that cost will *quintuple* by the year 2000 if current trends in health care coverage continue" (Henkoff 1991, p. 53). Italics in the original.

23   In a recent poll of America's CEOs (Chief Executive Officers) 63% indicated that escalating health care costs is one of their greatest problems. Of these same CEOs 69% did not think that the United States should adopt a nationalized health care system (Sheeline 1991, p. 58).

24   Another figure mentioned is that health care costs will "consume 17% of GNP by the year 2000 -- more than the current shares of education, defense, and recreation combined" (Smith 1991, p. 44).

25   Between May 15, 1991 and January 31, 1992, *JAMA (Journal of the American Medical Association)* published 13 articles on proposals for health care reform. Through August 1991 Congress considered some 20 proposals and bills on health care reform. The AMA, the American Association of Retired Persons, the American Hospital Association, and the National Leadership Coalition on Health Care all advanced proposals for health care reform. For a brief summary of these proposals see Blendon *et al*, (1992). For the AMA's response to national health care reform see Lundberg (1992).

26   When comparing health care expenditures among countries the most common measure used is the health-to-GDP ratio; that is, the "percent of a country's total output devoted to the health sector" (Schieber 1990, p. 159).

27   The latest figures for life expectancy in the United States demonstrate an improvement, at least for white males. The 1989 figures show that for all Americans life expectancy increased from 74.9 years in 1988 to 75.3 years in 1989. Black Americans, however, were not so fortunate. Their life expectancy decreased in 1989 to 64.8 years from 64.9 years

in 1988 (Center for Disease Control, 1992, pp. 1449-1450). Comparable Canadian figures are unavailable.

28 The latest U.S. figures indicate that the infant mortality rate has declined even further. In 1989 the infant mortality rate was listed at 9.8 deaths per 1,000 live births. As with life expectancy, the black infant mortality rate was significantly greater than the white infant mortality rate, 18.6 *versus* 8.1 deaths per 1,000 live births (Stout 1992b, p. B6). A recent study (Ropp *et al*, 1992, p. 2910) has concluded that in urban populations in the U.S., "with homicide as the leading or second leading cause of death in all age groups of black children, we have an epidemic."

29 Altman and Rodwin have argued that Americans don't have a "free market" in health insurance but rather only a "halfway competitive market" (Altman and Rodwin, 1988, p. 325). We shall return to this issue in Chapter VI.

30 It is estimated to have cost Americans "$95 each, out of their overall [1985 per capita expenditure for health care] $1,710" (Evans *et al*, 1989, p. 573).

31 It has been estimated, on the basis of international comparisons between Canada, the United States, and Britain expenditures for 1983, that in 1986 the United States could have reaped a savings, in terms of administrative costs, of $29.2 billion if it adopted a Canadian-style health care system, or $38.4 billion if the United States adopted a British style system (Himmelstein and Woolhandler, 1986, p. 443). In 1989, it was estimated that if Americans adopted a Canadian style system they would save in administrative costs "about $62 billion this year" (Woolhandler and Himmelstein, 1989, p. 2136).

32 Some have gone so far as to consider what would happen in the United States after NHI (national health insurance) has been implemented (Weil 1991). Others have advocated long-term care programs (Harrington *et al*, 1991). Others, sensing the inevitability of a NHI program (Lundberg 1992) have begun to specify the criteria that such a program should meet.

33 The most extensive and detailed documentation of the history of Canada's health care delivery system is that by Malcolm G. Taylor (1978 and 1987, 2nd ed.). The next best

overall source is Crichton *et al*, (1990), but some of her data are out of date.

34 Tommy Douglas, the leader of the CCF party, was elected as premier of the province in 1944 on a socialist platform the main part of which, as far as the electorate were concerned, was the promise of health care reform (Crichton *et al*, 1990, p. 161).

35 For a more detailed account of the changes that took place in Canada's health care system between 1974 and 1984, see Taylor (1986).

36 This Act is technically titled the Federal-Provincial Fiscal Arrangements and Federal Post-Secondary Education and Health Contribution Act but generally in the literature it is simply referred to as the Established Programs Financing Act or EPF Act (Crichton *et al*, 1990, p. 34).

37 Balance billing is the practice of physicians billing their patients for the difference between government fee schedules and what the physician actually wants for his service.

38 Coburn argues that the Canada Health Act was "yet another defeat for medicine and led directly to the doctor's strike in Ontario" (Coburn 1988, p. 106).

39 There have been three strikes by doctors in Canada, in Saskatchewan in 1962, in Quebec in 1970 (Crichton *et al*, 1990, pp. 175 and 33 respectively), and in Ontario in 1986. It is widely believed that Quebec's doctors went on strike to "preserve opting out and extra-billing" (Coburn 1988, p. 103). For an analysis of the Ontario doctor's strike see Stevenson *et al*, (1988).

40 That is, the number of hospitals as of 1984 (Crichton *et al*, 1990, p. 82).

41 The United States will soon implement a new national medicare fee schedule. This schedule will be based principally on a "resource-based relative value scale" (RBRVS). For a detailed analysis and comparison with how Canadian doctors are paid under Canada's health care system, see Rakich and Becker (1992).

42 Of the total health care expenditures in Canada in 1985, including non-medicare covered expenditures, public funds accounted for 75.9%. In the United States 41.1% of compa-

rable health care expenditures were publicly funded (Rakich 1991b, p. 29).

43 There are roughly 31 million Americans enrolled in Medicare and another 19 million are covered by Medicaid (Rakich 1991b, p. 27).

44 These figures might support some Canadians to joke that "President Bush needn't bother creating a kinder, gentler America, because it already exists. It's called Canada" (Kosterlitz 1989b, p. 1871).

45 All figures in this and the following paragraph are from Rakich (1991), pp. 25-42. I would also like to thank Professor Rakich for sending me this and related articles.

46 All the Canadian figures given below are 1989 figures, except for the figures for lithotripsy units and MRIs which are from 1988.

47 The third study has yet to be published and therefore we can only cite the anecdotal evidence provided by the media. "A study by Kenneth E. Thorpe of the University of North Carolina and colleagues show that while hospital administrative costs in California as a percentage of total operating expenses were 35% higher in 1985 than in New York, per-capita hospital costs were 17% *lower*. California is a competitive insurance market, while New York hospital fees are strictly regulated. The study found that California hospitals spend more on data processing and upper-level administrative jobs, areas associated with cost-control measures" (Winslow 1992, p. B1).

48 "The U.S. homicide rate has fluctuated between three and four times the Canadian rate for decades, and even greater differences are apparent for violent crimes more generally" (Hagan 1992, p. 127).

49 In Los Angeles County alone, during just the summer of 1987, there were 137 recorded incidents of roadway assaults using firearms; 39% of these involved just the "brandishing" of a firearm, while 61% were actual shootings (Onwuachi-Saunders *et al*, 1989, p. 2262). Incidents such as these are unheard of in Canada.

50 In 1983, in the United States, the leading cause of death among blacks aged 15 to 34 years was homicide. In 1986,

again in the United States, black males were 6 times more likely to die from a homicide than white males (Griffith and Bell, 1989, p. 2266). In fact, the U.S. Surgeon General just recently declared violence in America, especially violence due to firearms, was a "public health emergency" (Koop and Lundberg, 1992, p. 3075). No such comparable problem exists in Canada. For the most recent data on firearm related deaths and injuries, see the several related articles that appeared in *JAMA* 267:22 (June 12), 1992.

51 The most current estimates place the number of people in the United States suffering from AIDS or HIV at 205,000. This number is projected to increase, by 1995, to 240,000 to 335,000. The projected cost is expected to rise from the current $10.3 billion to $13.5 billion in 1995 (Chase 1992, p. B5). While Canada does have some AIDs patients, the percentage is nowhere near the U.S. figure.

52 The United States currently holds first place for divorce rates among seventeen western countries, and it has done so since at least 1961 and through until 1983. Canada, in 1961 was ranked 14th, and in 1983 was ranked 6th (Castles and Flood, 1991, p. 284).

53 There are an estimated 375,000 drug-exposed babies in the United States, while the problem is virtually negligible in Canada. The cost of treatment for the first five years is estimated at $35,000 per baby, or about $25 billion (Schwartz 1991, p. A10).

54 Daniels expanded on his argument to this problem in a later publication (Daniels 1988). Battin has argued, by extending Daniels' prudential lifespan argument, that people have a duty to die (Battin 1987).

55 Buchanan's notion of a "decent" minimum of health care is substantially different from a "just" minimum of health care. The former concept will be discussed in Chapter IV, while the latter will be explicated in Chapter VI.

56 For a critical examination of some of the initial problems Rawls' original argument faced see Daniels 1975; Nozick 1974, pp. 183-231. For more recent criticisms see the "Symposium on Rawlsian Theory of Justice: Recent Developiments" in *Ethics* 99:4 (July 1989). Thomas W. Pogge (1989) argues that Rawls' original work was, and still is, misunder-

stood by many of his critics. Kukathas and Pettit (1990) explicate Rawls' original work and attempt to identify the nature of its ongoing metamorphosis. In this latter regard see Rawls (1988, 1987, 1985, and 1982).

57 The rights Daniels has been arguing in favor of -- and what Buchanan will be arguing in favor of in the next chapter -- are not the same as the rights that are typically defended by libertarians, the rights to life, liberty and property. On the contrary they are much more like the positive rights we identified in Chapter 1, or what Charles Reich called, in his seminal article on the subject, "the new property" (Reich 1964, 1965); that is, entitlements to different forms of government-created wealth and largess. Also see Van Alstyne (1977), and Melnick (1990).

58 See Daniels (1983) for his response to Stern's criticisms.

59 This is not to say that people who do not file claims have not benefitted from having insurance, for they have. Those people who have not filed claims will have received the benefit of having been protected against the risks of becoming sick and/or injured.

60 Kenneth Arrow argues that the ignorance we face with respect to the outcome of treatment, as well the ignorance we face with respect to the incidence of disease, is the main reason for justifying the medical profession's monopoly on the practice of medicine. We explicate and criticize Arrow's argument in Chapter VI.

61 It is estimated that more than 1 million young people start to smoke every year, thus increasing U.S. health care expenditures by $9 to $10 billion (in 1990 dollars discounted at 3%) over the course of their lifetime (Hodgson 1992, p. 111).

62 Some have argued that the marginal costs for the sixth test have been underestimated by over $110 million (Prescott *et al*, 1980, p. 1306), while others have argued that the results were overestimated by almost the complete $47 million (Brown *et al*, 1991, p. 440). For Neuhauser's response to both of these charges see, respectively, Neuhauser (1980) and (1990).

63 We shall return to the issue of restricting people's liberty in

Chapter VI, for it plays a crucial role in our argument for a just minimum of health care.

64 Buchanan and Stern make a similar point with respect to Daniels' claim that health care institutions have the "limited function of maintaining normal species functioning" (Daniels 1985, p. 53). *Cf* Buchanan (1984), p. 63 and Stern (1983), p. 346.

65 I am indebted to Loren Lomasky for this particular example.

66 The assumption that a collective effort to establish a decent minimum of health is a more important form of beneficence than individual charitable acts is a tendentious assumption and thus needs to be substantiated. However, *ad arguendo*, we shall grant Buchanan the assumption and still demonstrate that his arguments are invalid.

67 *Cf* James Buchanan's (1968) *The Demand and Supply of Public Goods*.

68 *Cf* McKinlay and McKinlay, (1977), p. 414, italics in the original.

69 The report does not allow one to determine how much of these charitable contributions were donated to religious organizations.

70 For a fuller account of this report see "Giving USA," which is available from the AAFRC Trust for Philanthropy, 25 West 43rd Street, New York, NY, 10036.

71 For earlier versions of the arguments which led up to *Morals By Agreement* see Gauthier (1990).

72 The assumption that people do not take an interest in the interests of others is contrary to fact, for people do take an interest in the interests of others. The interest we have in other's interests can be either a positive interest or a negative interest. Peter Vallentyne argues that this counterfactual assumption raises a difficulty for Gauthier's argument at the outset. *Cf* Vallentyne (1991), pp. 71-75.

73 For an account of an argument in favor of an actual agreement, see Gilbert Harman (1983) "Justice and Moral Bargaining."

74 Christopher Morris argues that Gauthier's theory can take into account those who cannot contribute to the cooperative

enterprise. Morris draws a distinction between primary and secondary moral standing and argues that those who do not have primary moral standing, animals, defective newborns and the like, might piggyback on some who do have primary moral standing if those who do have primary moral standing are concerned about the latter's interests. *Cf* Morris (1991).

75 With regard to bargaining being cost free, Robert Sugden argues that if it is cost free, then there is no reason to reach agreement. *Cf* Sugden (1990).

76 Recall also Reinhardt similar observation. "In any given year, some 70 to 80% of health care expenditures tend to be caused by only about 10% of the population" (Reinhardt 1987, p. 169).

Bibliography

Abelson, Julia. 1992. "An Overview of the Development of Canada's Health Care System," unpublished manuscript presented to the Fifth Annual Reddin Symposium at Bowling Green State University on January 18, 1992.

AMA Council on Ethical and Judicial Affairs, 1992. "Conflicts of Interest: Physician Ownership of Medical Facilities," *Journal of the American Medical Association* 267:17 (May 6), pp. 2366-2369.

"Americans Donated $104 Billion in '88," 1989. *New York Times* (June 7), p. A16.

Anderson, Jack and Dale Van Atta. 1991. "Doctor Owned Labs Test Profit Motive," *Washington Post* (Monday, August 5), Section D, p. 8.

Anderson, Jane. 1992. "Health Costs Cited as Major Problem," *Medical Tribune* (Monday, June 25), p. 7.

Alma-Ata Declaration. The Declaration of Alma-Ata is reprinted in full in Halfdan Mahler's "The Meaning of 'health for all by the year 2000'," *World Health Forum* 2:1 (1981) pp. 21-22.

Altman, Lawrence K. 1992. "Surgical Injuries Lead to New Rules," *New York Times* (Sunday, June 14), p. 1.

Altman, Stuart H., and Marc A. Rodwin. 1988. "Halfway Competitive Markets and Ineffective Regulation: The American Health Care System," *Journal of Health Politics, Policy and Law* 13:2 (Summer), pp. 323-339.

Andrews, Lori B. 1986. *Deregulating Doctors: Do Medical Licensing Laws Meet Today's Health Care Needs?* Emmaus, PA: People's Medical Society.

Arrow, Kenneth. 1981. "Gifts and Exchanges," *Medicine and*

Moral Philosophy (ed. Cohen, Nagel, and Scanlon). Princeton: Princeton University Press, pp. 139-158

___. 1973. "Some Ordinalist-Utilitarian Notes on Rawls' Theory of Justice," *Journal of Philosophy* 70:9 (May 10), pp. 245-263

___. 1963. "Uncertainty and the Welfare Economics of Medical Care," *American Economic Review* 53:5 (December) pp. 941-973.

Barer, Morris L. 1991. "Controlling Medical Costs in Canada," *Journal of the American Medical Association* 265:18 (May 8), pp. 2392-2394.

___. 1988. "Regulating Physician Supply: The Evolution of British Columbia's Bill 41," *Journal of Health Politics, Policy and Law* 13:1 (Spring), pp. 1-25.

Barer, Morris L., and Robert G. Evans. 1992. "Interpreting Canada: Models, Mind-Sets and Myths," *Health Affairs* 11:1 (Spring), pp. 44-61.

___. 1986. "Riding North on a South-Bound Horse? Expenditures, Prices, Utilization and Incomes in the Canadian Health Care System," *Medicare at Maturity: Achievements, Lessons and Challenges* (eds. Evans and Stoddart). Calgary: The University of Calgary Press, pp. 53-163.

Barer, Morris L., Robert G. Evans, and Roberta J. Labelle. 1988. "Fee Controls as Cost Controls: Tales From the Frozen North," *The Milbank Quarterly* 66:1, pp. 1-64.

Barnes, John A. 1990. "Canadian Cross Border to Save Their Lives," *Wall Street Journal* (Wednesday, December 12), p. A16.

Barron, Donna. 1992. "The World of CD-ROM," *Physicians and Computers* 10:2 (June) pp. 20-27.

Battin, Margaret P. 1987. "Age Rationing and the Just Distribution of Health Care: Is There a Duty to Die?" *Ethics* 97 (January), pp. 317-340.

Barnhill, William. 1992. "Canadian Health Care: Would It Work Here?," *Arthritis Today* (November/December), pp. 35-44.

"B.C. Doctors Looking to Emigrate to the U.S.," 1992. *Globe and Mail* (Friday, May 8), p. A4.

Beauchamp, Tom L and Laurence B. McCullough. 1984. *Medical Ethics: The Moral Responsibility of Physicians*. Englewood Cliffs, N.J.: Prentice-Hall, Inc.

Beck, Joan. 1985a. "Doctors, Money and Health," *Chicago Tribune* (January 28), Section 1, p. 14.

_____. 1985b. "Please Don't Leave This Around," *Chicago Tribune* (March 11), Section 1, p. 12.

Benham, Lee and Alexandra Benham. 1975a. "Regulating Through the Professions: A Perspective on Information Control," *Journal of Law and Economics* 28:2 (October), pp. 421-447.

_____. 1975b. "The Impact of Incremental Medical Services on Health Status, 1963-1970," *Equity in Health Services: Empirical Analyses in Social Policy* (eds. Anderson, Kravitz, and Anderson). Cambridge, MA: Ballinger Publishing Company.

Bennett, William J. 1992. "The Moral Origin of the Urban Crisis," *Wall Street Journal* (Friday, May 8), p. 14.

Berenson, Robert and John Holahan. 1992. "Sources of the Growth in Medicare Physician Expenditures," *Journal of the American Medical Association* 267:5 (February 5), pp. 687-691.

Birch, Stephen. 1988. "The Identification of Supplier-Inducement in a Fixed Price System of Health Care Provision: The Case of Dentistry in the United Kingdom," *Journal of Health Economics* 7, pp. 129-150.

Blendon, Robert J., Jennifer N. Edwards, and Andrew L. Hyams. 1992. "Making the Critical Choices," *Journal of the American Medical Association* 267:18 (May 13), pp. 2509-2520.

Blendon, Robert J., R. Leitman, I. Morrison, and K. Donelan. 1990. "Satisfaction with Health Care Systems in Ten Nations," *Health Affairs* 9:2, pp. 185-192.

Blendon, Robert J. and Humphrey Taylor. 1989. "Views on Health Care in Three Nations," *Health Affairs* 8:1 (Spring), pp. 149-157.

Bloom, Paul N. and Ronald Stiff. 1980. "Advertising and Health Care Professions," *Journal of Health Politics, Policy and Law* 4:4 (Winter), pp. 642-665.

Blumberg, Mark S. 1988. "Measuring Surgical Quality in Maryland: A Model," *Health Affairs* 7:1 (Spring), pp. 62-78.

Blumstein, James F. and Michael Zubkoff. 1979. "Public Choice in Health: Problems, Politics and Perspectives on Formulating National Health Policy," *Journal of Health Politics, Policy and Law* 4:3 (Fall), pp. 382-413.

Boorse, Christopher. 1981. "On the Distinction Between Disease and Illness," *Medicine and Moral Philosophy: A Phi-*

losophy & Public Affairs Reader (eds. Cohen, Nagel, and Scanlon). Princeton: Princeton University Press, pp. 3-22.

Brahams, Diana. 1989. "Frauds on the Public," *Lancet* (October 14), pp. 929-931.

Brandt, Richard B. 1983. "The Concept of a Moral Right," *Journal of Philosophy* 80, pp. 29-45.

Brennan, Troyen A., Liesi E. Hebert, Nan M. Laird, Ann Lawthers, Kenneth E. Thorpe, Luian L. Leape, A. Russell Localio, Stuart R. Lipsitz, Joseph P. Newhouse, Paul C. Weiler, and Howard H. Hiatt. 1991. "Hospital Characteristics Associated With Adverse Events and Substandard Care," *Journal of the American Medical Association* 265:24 (June 26), pp. 3265-3269.

Brennan, Troyen A., Lucian L. Leape, Nan M. Laird, Liesi Hebert, A. Russell Localio, Ann G. Lawthers, Joseph P. Newhouse, Paul C. Weiler, and Howard H. Hiatt. 1991. "Incidence of Adverse Events and Negligence in Hospitalized Patients: Results of the Harvard Medical Practice Study I," *New England Journal of Medicine* 324:6 (February 7), pp. 370-376.

Brown, E. Richard. 1979. *Rockefeller Medicine Men: Medicine and Capitalism in America.* Berkeley: University of California Press, 1979.

Brown, Lawrence D. 1990. "The Medically Uninsured: Problems, Policies, and Politics," *Journal of Health Politics, Policy and Law* 15:2 (Summer), pp. 413-426.

Brown, Kaye and Colin Burrows. 1990. "The Sixth Stool Guiac Test: $47 Million That Never Was," *Journal of Health Economics* 9, pp. 429-445.

Buchanan, Allen. 1984. "The Right to a Decent Minimum of Health Care" *Philosophy & Public Affairs* 13:1 (Winter), pp. 55-78.

___. 1983. "The Right to a Decent Minimum of Health Care," *Securing Access to Health Care.* Washington: U.S. Government Printing Office, pp. 207-238.

Buchanan, Allen E. and Dan W. Brock. 1989. *Deciding for Others.* Cambridge: Cambridge University Press.

Buchanan, James M. 1968. T*he Demand and Supply of Public Goods.* Chicago: Rand McNally & Company.

Bunker, John P. 1970. "A Comparison of Operations and Surgeons in the United States and in England and Wales," *New England Journal of Medicine* 282:3 (January 15), pp. 135-144.

Burstein, Philip L. and Jerry Cromwell. 1985. "Relative

Incomes and Rates of Return for Physicians," *Journal of Health Economics* 4:1 (March), pp. 63-78.

Burton, Thomas M. 1992. "Physicians Who Own Labs May Refer Patients to Them for Tests, AMA Says," *Wall Street Journal* (Wednesday, June 24), p. B12.

Cangello, Vincent W. 1992. "The Uninsured Problem: Not as Big as We're Told," *Private Practice* 24:7 (July), pp. 30-31.

Castles, Francis G. and Michael Flood. 1991. "Divorce, the Law and Social Context: Families of National and the Legal Dissolution of Marriage," *Acta Sociologica* 34:4, pp. 279-297.

Center for Disease Control. 1992. "Mortality Patterns - United States, 1989," *Journal of the American Medical Association* 267:11 (March 18), pp. 1449-1450.

Chase, Marilyn. 1992. "U.S. Forecasts Growth in Cases of AIDS, HIV," *Wall Street Journal* (Monday, July 20), p. B5.

Clark, Nicola. 1992. "View From the Forum," *Cortlandt Forum* 5:7 (July), pp. 19-22.

Coburn, David. 1988. "Canadian Medicine: Dominance or Proletarianization," *The Milbank Quarterly* 66:Supp. 2, pp. 92-116.

Cohen, Harris S. 1980. "On Professional Power and Conflict of Interest: State Licensing Boards on Trial," *Journal of Health Politics, Policy and Law* 5:2 (Summer), pp. 291-308.

Coleman, Jules. 1992. *Risks and Wrongs.* Cambridge: Cambridge University Press.

Contandriopoulos. Andre-Pierre. 1986. "Cost Containment Through Payment Mechanisms; The Quebec Experience," *Journal of Public Health Policy* 72, pp. 224-238.

Coombs, Robert H. and Pauline S. Powers. 1985. "Socialization for Death," *Urban Life* 4:3 (October), pp. 250-271.

Cornes, Richard and Todd Sandler. 1986. *The Theory of Externalities, Public Goods, and Club Goods.* Cambridge: Cambridge University Press.

Coyte, Peter C., Donald N. Dewes, and Michael J. Trebilcock. 1991. "Canadian Medical Malpractice Liability: An Empirical Analysis of Recent Trends," *Journal of Health Economics* 10, pp. 143-168.

Crane, Thomas S. 1992. "The Problem of Physician Self-referral Under the Medicare and Medicaid Antikickback Statute," *Journal of the American Medical Association* 268:1 (July 1), pp. 85-91.

Crawley, Robert, Richard Belsey, Darrell Brock, and Daniel M. Baer. 1986. "Regulation of Physician' Office Laboratories," *Journal of the American Medical Association* 255:3 (January 17), pp. 374- 382.

Crenshaw, Albert B. 1991. "Diagnosing Medical Fraud: Cheaters are Increasingly Doctors, Clinics, Other Providers," *Washington Post* (June 16), Section H, p. 3.

Crichton, Anne, David Hsu, and (with the assistance of) Stella Tsang. 1990. *Canada's Health Care System: Its Funding and Organization*. Ottawa: Canadian Hospital Association Press.

Cromwell, Jerry and Janet B. Mitchell. 1986. "Physician-Induced Demand for Surgery," *Journal of Health Economics* 5:4 (December), pp. 293-313.

Cust, Kenneth F.T. 1991. "Hypothetical Contractarianism and the Disclosure Requirement Problem in Informed Consent," *Journal of Medical Humanities* 12:3, pp. 119-138.

Daniels, Norman. 1988. *Am I My Parent's Keeper?: An Essay on Justice Between the Young and the Old*. Oxford: Oxford University Press.

___. 1985. *Just Health Care*. Cambridge: Cambridge University Press.

___. (ed.). 1975. *Reading Rawls*. New York: Basic Books.

___. 1983. "A Reply to Some Stern Criticisms and a Remark on Health Care Rights" *Journal of Medicine and Philosophy* 8:4 (November 1983), pp. 363-371.

Danzon, Patricia M. 1992. "Hidden Overhead Costs: Is Canada's System Really Less Expensive?" *Health Affairs* 11:1 (Spring), pp. 21-43.

___. 1991. "Liability for Medical Malpractice," *Journal of Economic Perspectives* 5:3 (Summer), pp. 51-69.

Dardanoni, Valentine and Adam Wagstaff. 1990. "Uncertainty and the Demand for Medical Care," *Journal of Health Economics* 9, pp. 23-38.

de Jasay, Anthony. 1989. *Social Contract, Free Ride: A Study of the Public Goods Problem*. Oxford: Clarendon Press.

Desmeules, Marie and Robert Semenciw. 1991. "The Impact of Medical Care On Mortality in Canada, 1958-1988," Canadian *Journal of Public Health* 82:3 (May/June), pp. 209-211.

"Doctors' Strike Lowered the Death Rate." 1978. *Science News* 114:18 (October 28), p. 293.

Diffy, Maureen Nevin. 1990. "Survey of Corporate Contributions," *The Conference Board* pp. 1-60.

Doebbeling, Bradley N., Gail S. Stanley, Carol T. Sheetz, Michael A. Pfaller, Alison K. Houston, Linda Ammis, Ning Li, and Richard P. Wenzel. 1992. "Comparative Efficacy of Alternative Hand-Washing Agents in Reducing Nosocomial Infections in Intensive Care Units," *New England Journal of Medicine* 327:2 (July 9), pp. 88-93.

Donaldson, Robert M. 1992. "Computers at the Bedside," *Cortlandt Forum* 5:11 (November), p. 48cc.

Dranove, David. "The Costs of Compliance With the 1962 FDA Amendments," *Journal of Health Economics* 10, pp. 235-238.

Dworkin, Gerald. 1982. "Is More Choice Better Than Less?" *Midwest Studies in Philosophy* Vol. VII (ed. French, Uehling, and Wettstein). Minneapolis: University of Minnesota Press, pp. 47-61.

Eastman, Peggy. 1992. "Regulating Physician Office Labs," *Geriatric Consultant* 11:1 (July/August), pp. 13-15.

"Elective Surgery: Cut it Out." 1979. *Science News* 115:1 (January 6), p. 9.

Engelhardt, H. Tristram, Jr. 1991. *Bioethics and Secular Humanism*. Philadelphia: Trinity Press International.

____. 1986. *The Foundations of Bioethics*. New York: Oxford University Press.

____. 1981. "Health Care Allocation: Response to the Unjust, Unfortunate, and the Undesirable," *Justice and Health Care* (e.d Shelp). Dordrecht: D. Reidel Publishing Co., pp. 121-137.

Enthoven, Alain. 1988. "Managed Competition of Alternative Delivery Systems," *Journal of Health Politics, Policy and Law* 13:2 (Summer), pp. 305-321.

Epstein, Richard A. 1992. *Forbidden Grounds: The Case Against Employment Discrimination Laws*. Cambridge: Harvard University Press.

Evans, Robert G. 1991. "Advanced Medical Technology and Elderly People," *Too Old For Health Care?* (eds. Binstock and Post). Baltimore: The Johns Hopkins University Press, pp. 44-74.

____. 1988. "Split Visions: Interpreting Cross-Border Differences in Health Spending," *Health Affairs* 7:5 (Winter), pp. 17-24.

Evans, Robert G., Jonathan Lomas, Morris L. Barer, Roberta J. Labelle, Catherine Fooks, Gregory L. Stoddart, Geoffrey M. Anderson, David Feeny, Amiram Gafni, George Torrance, and William G. Tholl. 1989. "Controlling Health Expenditures: The Canadian Reality," *New England Journal of Medicine* 320:9 (March 2), pp. 571-577.

Faden, Ruth R. and Tom L. Beauchamp. 1986. *A History and Theory of Informed Consent.* Oxford: Oxford University Press.

Farley, Pamela J. 1986. "Theories of the Price and Quantity of Physician Services: A Synthesis and Critique," *Journal of Health Economics* 5:4 (December), pp. 315-333.

Farnsworth, Clyde H. 1992. "Canada Rethinks its Health Care," *New York Times* (November 24), p. 9.

Feinberg, Joel. 1970. "The Nature and Value of Rights," *Journal of Value Inquiry* 4:4 (Winter), pp. 243-257.

Feldman, Roger. 1988. "Competition Among Physicians, Revisited," *Journal of Health Politics, Policy and Law* 13:2 (Summer), pp. 239-261.

Feldman, Roger and Michael A. Morrisey. 1990. "Health Economics: A Report From the Field," *Journal of Health Politics, Policy and Law* 15:3 (Fall), pp. 627-646.

Feldman, Roger and Roger Sloan. 1989. "Reply From Feldman and Sloan," *Journal of Health Politics, Policy and Law* 14:3 (Fall), pp. 621-625.

Ferguson, Tom. 1992. "Patient, Heal Thyself," *The Futurist* 76:1 (Jan/Feb), pp. 9-13.

Fischer, Anne B. 1992. "The New Debate Over The Very Rich," *Fortune* 125:13 (June 29), pp. 42-54.

"Fraud Seen Accounting for 10% of Healthcare Spending." 1992. *Physician Financial News* 10:12 (June 30), p. 12.

Fried, Charles. 1978. *Right and Wrong.* Cambridge, MA: Harvard University Press.

Friedman, Milton. 1962. *Capitalism and Freedom.* Chicago: University of Chicago Press.

Friedson, Eliot. 1986. *Professional Powers.* Chicago: University of Chicago Press.

Fuchs, Victor R. 1988. "Learning From the Canadian Experience," *Health Affairs* 7:5 (Winter), pp. 25-30.

___. 1978. "The Supply of Surgeons and the Demand for Operations," *Journal of Human Resources* 13:Supp., pp. 35-56.

___. 1974. "Some Economic Aspects of Mortality in Developed Countries," *Economics of Health and Medical Care* (ed. Perlman). New York: John Wiley & Sons, pp. 174-193.

Fuchs, Victor R., and James S. Hahn. 1990. "How Does Canada Do It: A Comparison of Expenditures for Physician's Services in the United States and Canada," *New England Journal of Medicine* 323:13 (September 27), pp. 884-890.

Fulford, K.W.M. 1989. *Moral Theory and Medical Practice*. Cambridge: Cambridge University Press.

Gabel, Jon R., Howard Cohen, and Steven Fink. 1989. "American Views on Health Care: Foolish Inconsistencies," *Health Affairs* 8:1 (Spring), pp. 103-118.

Gabel, Jon R. and Jonathan H. Rice. 1985. "Reducing Public Expenditures for Physician Services: The Price of Paying Less," *Journal of Health Politics, Policy and Law* 9:4 (Winter), pp. 595-609.

Gagner, Natalie. 1992a. "Surgical Fees Growing," *American Medical News* (July 6/13), p. 33.

___. 1992b. "Sign of the Times," *American Medical News* (July 6/13), p. 33.

___. 1992c. "Where Does The Medical Dollar Go?" *American Medical News* (July 20), p. 26.

Garcia, James L. 1989. "Fraud: The Hidden Elements of Health Care Costs," *Compensation and Benefits Management* (August), pp. 49-51.

Gaus, Gerald F. 1990. *Value and Justification: The Foundations of Liberal Theory*. Cambridge: Cambridge University Press.

Gauthier, David. 1991. "Rational Constraint: Some Last Words," *Contractarianism and Rational Choice: Essays on David Gauthier's Morals By Agreement* (ed. Vallentyne). New York: Cambridge University Press. pp. 323-330.

___. 1990. *Moral Dealing: Contract, Ethics, and Reason*. Ithaca: Cornell University Press.

___. 1988. "Morality, Rational Choice, and Semantic Representation: A Reply to My Critics," *Social Philosophy & Policy* 5:2 (Spring 1988) pp. 173-221.

___. 1986. *Morals By Agreement*. Oxford: Clarendon Press.

General Accounting Office. 1991. *Canadian Health Insurance: Lessons for the United States*. Washington, D.C.

Gibson, Robert M. 1979. "National Health Expenditures," *Health Care Financing Review* (Summer), pp. 1-36.

Goodman, John C. 1992. *How the Federal Government is Causing Our Nation's Health Care Crisis.* (NCPA Policy Report No. 119). Dallas: National Center for Policy Analysis.

_____. 1980. *The Regulation of Medical Care: Is the Price Too High?.* San Francisco: CATO Institute.

Goodman, John C. and Gerald L. Musgrave. 1991. *Twenty Myths About National Health Care Insurance* (NCPA Policy Report No. 128). Dallas: National Center for Policy Analysis.

Green, Jerry. 1987. "Physician-Induced Demand for Medical Care," *Journal of Human Resources* 13:Supp., pp. 21-34.

Griffith, Ezra E. H., and Carl C. Bell. 1989. "Recent Trends in Suicide and Homicide Among Blacks," *Journal of the American Medical Association* 262:16 (October 27), pp. 2265-2269.

Grumbach, Kevin and Philip R. Lee. 1991. "How Many Physicians Can We Afford?" *Journal of the American Medical Association* 265:18 (May 8), pp. 2369-2372.

Grytten, Jostein, Dorthe Holst, and Petter Laake. 1990. "Supplier Inducement: Its Effect on Dental Services in Norway," *Journal of Health Economics* 9, pp. 483-491.

Hadley, Elizabeth Harrison. 1989. "Nurses and Prescriptive Authority: A Legal and Economic Analysis," *American Journal of Law and Medicine* 15:2/3, pp. 245-299.

Hafferty, Frederic W. 1988. "Theories at the Crossroads," *The Milbank Quarterly* 66:Supp., pp. 202-225.

Hagan, John. 1992. "Class Fortification Against Crime in Canada," *Canadian Review of Sociology and Anthropology* 29:2 (May), pp. 126-139.

Haislmaier, Edmond F. 1991. "Northern Discomfort: The Ills of the Canadian Health System," *Policy Review* 58 (Fall), pp. 32-37.

Hamowy, Ronald. 1979. "The Early Development of Medical Licensing Laws in the United States, 1875-1900," *Journal of Libertarian Studies* 3:1, pp. 73-119.

_____. 1984. *Canadian Medicine: A Study in Restricted Entry.* Vancouver: The Fraser Institute.

Hampton, Jean. 1987. "Free-Rider Problems in the Production of Collective Goods," *Economics and Philosophy* 3, pp. 245-273.

Harman, Gilbert. 1983. "Justice and Moral Bargaining," *Social Philosophy and Policy* 1, pp. 114-131.

Harrington, Charlene, Christine Cassel, Carrol L. Estes, Steffie Woolhandler, David U. Himmelstein, and the Working Group on Long-Term Care Program Design. 1991. "A National Long-Term Care Program for the United States," *Journal of the American Medical Association* 266:21 (December 4), pp. 3023-3029.

Harrison, Michael. 1992. "New Teaching Tools Help Students Stay 'Anatomically Correct'," *Advance* (Summer) pp. 16-19.

Hartwell, R. M. 1974. "The Economic History of Medical Care," *The Economics of Health and Medical Care* (ed. Perlman). New York: John Wiley & Sons, pp. 3-20.

Haug, Marie R. 1988. "A Re-examination of the Hypothesis of Physician Deprofessionalization," *The Milbank Quarterly* 66:Supp. 2, pp. 48-56.

Henkoff, Ronald. 1991. "Yes, Companies Can Cut Health Costs," *Fortune* (July 1) pp. 52-56.

Hiatt, Howard H., Benjamin J. Barnes, Troyen A Brennan, Nan M. Liard, Ann G. Lawthers, Lucian L. Leape, A. Russell Localio, Joseph P. Newhouse, Lynn M. Peterson, Kenneth E. Thorpe, Paul C. Weiler, and William G. Johnson. 1989. "A Study of Medical Injury and Medical Malpractice: An Overview," *New England Journal of Medicine* 321:7 (August 17), pp. 480-484.

Hillman, Bruce J. and Catherine A. Joseph, Michael R. Mabry, Jonathan H. Sunshine, Stephen D. Kennedy, and Monica Noether. 1990. "Frequency and Costs of Diagnostic Imaging in Office Practice -- A Comparison of Self-Referring and Radiologist-Referring Physicians," *New England Journal of Medicine* 323:23 (December 6), pp. 1604-1608.

Hillman, Bruce J. and George T. Olsen, Patricia E. Griffith, Jonathan H. Sunshine, Catherine A. Joseph, Stephen D. Kennedy, William R. Nelson, and Lee B. Bernhardt. 1992. "Physicians' Utilization and Charges for Outpatient Diagnostic Imaging in a Medicare Population," *Journal of the American Medical Association* 268:15 (October 21), pp. 2050-2054.

Himmelstein, David U. and Steffie Woolhandler. 1986. "Cost Without Benefit: Administrative Waste in U.S. Health Care," *New England Journal of Medicine* 314:7 (February 13), pp. 441-445.

Hobbes, Thomas. 1988. *Leviathan* (ed. Macpherson). London: Penguin Books.

Hodgson, Thomas A. 1992. "Cigarette Smoking and Lifetime Medical Expenditures," *The Milbank Quarterly* 7:1, pp. 81-125.

Hohfeld, Wesley. 1919. *Fundamental Legal Conceptions As Applied in Judicial Reasoning* (ed. Walter Wheeler Cook). New Haven: Yale University Press.

Hughes, John S. 1991. "How Well Has Canada Contained the Costs of Doctoring?" *Journal of the American Medical Association* 265:18 (May 8), pp. 2347-2351.

Hugick, Larry and Graham Hueber. 1991. "Pharmacists and Clergy Rate Highest for Honesty and Ethics," *Gallop Poll Monthly* (May), pp. 29-31.

Iglehart, J.K. 1986a. "Canada's Health Care System I," *New England Journal of Medicine* 315:3, pp. 202-208.

____. 1986b. "Canada's Health Care System II," *New England Journal of Medicine* 315:12, pp. 778-784.

____. 1986c. "Canada's Health Care System III: Addressing the Problem of Physician Supply," *New England Journal of Medicine* 315:25, pp. 202-208.

Inlander, Charles B., Lowell S. Levin, and Ed Weiner. 1988. *Medicine on Trial.* New York: Pantheon Books.

"Insurance Fraud Usually Not Spotted, Report Says," 1992. *Family Practice News* 22:13 (July 1), p. 41.

In the matter of Karen Quinlan, 70 N.J. 10, 355 A. 2d. 647.

Jajich-Toth, Cindy and Burns W. Roper. 1990. "American Views on Health Care: A Study in Contradictions," *Health Affairs* 9:4 (Winter), pp. 149-157.

Jesilow, Paul, Gilber Geis, and Henry Pontell. 1991. "Fraud by Physicians Against Medicaid," *Journal of the American Medical Association* 266:23 (December 18), pp. 3318-3322.

Johnson, William G., Troyen A. Brennan, Joseph P. Newhouse, Lucian L. Leape, Ann G. Lawthers, Howard H. Hiatt, and Paul C. Weiler. 1992. "The Economic Consequences of Medical Injuries," *Journal of the American Medical Association* 267:18 (May 13), pp. 2487-2492.

Kalish, Susan. 1992. "Jobs and Health Insurance: The Link Weakens," *Population Today* 20:5 (May), pp. 8-9.

Kelly, Karla. 1985. "Nurse Practitioner Challenges to the Orthodox Structure of Health Care Delivery: Regulation and Restraints on Trade," *American Journal of Law and Medicine* 11:2, pp. 195-225.

Kessel, Reuben A. 1975. "Price Discrimination in Medicine,"

Microeconomics: Selected Readings, 2nd ed., (ed. Mansfield) NY: W.W. Norton and Co., Inc., pp. 272-291.

Koop, Everett C., and George D. Lundberg. 1992. "Violence in America: A Public Health Emergency," *Journal of the American Medical Association* 267:22 (June 10), pp. 3075-3076.

Kosterlitz, Julie. 1989a. "Taking Care of Canada: Part 1," *National Journal* 21:28 (July 15), pp. 1792-1797.

___. 1989b. "But Not For Us?: Part 2," *National Journal* 21:29 (July 22), pp. 1871-1875.

Kotulak, Ronald. 1985. "Nation's Doctors in Deep Trouble," *Chicago Tribune* (May 28), Section 2, p. 4.

Kraus, Jody and Jules Coleman. 1987. "Morality and the Theory of Rational Choice," *Ethics* 97:4 (July), pp. 715-749.

Kukathas, Chandran and Philip Pettit. 1990. *Rawls: A Theory of Justice and its Critics*. Cambridge, UK: Polity Press.

Law, Maureen and Jean Lariviere. 1988. "Canada and WHO: Giving and Receiving," *Health Promotion* 26:4 (Spring), pp. 2-8 and p. 16.

Lazenby, Helen C. and Suzanne W. Letsch. 1990. "National Health Expenditures, 1989," *Health Care Financing Review* 12:2 (Winter), pp. 1-26.

Leape, Lucian L., Troyen A. Brennan, Nan Laird, Ann G. Lawthers, A. Russell Localio, Benjamin A. Barnes, Liesi Hebert, Joseph P. Newhouse, Paul C. Weiler, and Howard Hiatt. 1991. "The Nature of Adverse Events in Hospitalized Patients: Results of the Harvard Medical Practice Study II," *New England Journal of Medicine* 324:6 (February 7), pp. 377-384.

Lees, Dennis S. and Robert G. Rice. 1965. "Uncertainty and the Welfare Economics of Medical Care: Commentary," *The American Economic Review* 55:1 (March), pp. 140-154.

LeRoy, Lauren. 1982. "The Cost-Effectiveness of Nurse Practitioners," *Nursing in the 1980s: Crises, Opportunities, Challenges* (ed. Aiken). Philadelphia: J.B. Lippincott Co., pp. 295-314.

Levit, Katherine R. and Cathy A. Cowan. 1991a. "Business, Households, and Governments: Health Care Costs, 1990," *Health Care Financing Review* 13:2 (Winter), pp. 83-93.

Levit, Katherine R., Helen C. Lazenby, Cathy A. Cowan, and Suzanne W. Letsch. 1991b. "National Health Expenditures, 1990," *Health Care Financing Review* 13:1 (Fall), pp. 29-54.

Lewit, Eugene M. 1986. "The Diffusion of Surgical Technology: Who's On First?" *Journal of Health Economics* 5:1 (March), pp. 99- 102.

Light, Donald and Sol Levine. 1988. "The Changing Character of the Medical Profession: A Theoretical Overview," *The Milbank Quarterly* 66:Supp. 2, pp. 10-32.

Lindsay, Cotton M., Steven Honda and Benjamin Zycher. 1978. *Canada's National Health Insurance: Lessons for the United States*. Roche Laboratories.

Localio, A. Russell, Ann G. Lawthers, Troyen A. Brennan, Nan M. Laird, Liesi E. Hebert, Lynn M. Peterson, Joseph P. Newhouse, Paul C. Weiler, and Howard H. Hiatt. 1991. "Relation Between Malpractice Claims and Adverse Events Due to Negligence: Results of the Harvard Medical Practice Study III," *New England Journal of Medicine* 325:4 (July 25), pp. 245-251.

Locke, John. 1965. *Two Treatises of Government* (ed. Laslett). Cambridge: Cambridge University Press.

Lomas, Jonathan, Catherine Fooks, Thomas H. Rice, Roberta J. Labelle. 1989. "Paying Physicians in Canada: Minding Our P's and Q's," *Health Affairs* 8:1 (Spring), pp. 80-102.

Lomasky, Loren. 1987. *Persons, Rights, and the Moral Community*. New York: Oxford University Press.

___. 1981. "Medical Progress and National Health Care," *Medicine and Moral Philosophy* (ed. by Cohen, Nagel, and Scanlon). Princeton: Princeton University Press, 1981, pp. 115-138.

Lundberg, George D. 1992. "National Health Care Reform: The Aura of Inevitability Intensifies," *Journal of the American Medical Association* 267:18 (May 13), pp. 2521-2524.

Mahler, Halfdan. 1981. "The Meaning of 'health for all by the year 2000'," *World Health Forum* 2:1, pp. 5-22.

Manson, JoAnn E., Heather Tosteson, Paul M. Ridker, Suzanne Satterfield, Patricia Hebert, Gerald T. O'Connor, Julie E. Buring, and Charles H. Hennekens. 1992. "The Primary Prevention of Myocardial Infarction," *New England Journal of Medicine* 326:21 (May 21), pp. 1406-1416.

Markowitz, Gerald E. and David Karl Rosner. 1973. "Doctors in Crisis: A Study of the Use of Medical Education Reform to Establish Modern Professional Elitism in Medicine," *American Quarterly* 25:1 (March), pp. 83-107.

Matas, Robert. 1992. "Doctors Winning PR Battle," *The Globe and Mail* (Tuesday, January 5), p. A1-A2.

148 *A Just Minimum of Health Care*

McCormick, Brian. 1992. "Referral Ban Softened," *American Medical News* (July 6/13), p. 1 and p. 92.

McDowell, Jr., Theodore N. 1989. "Physician Self-Referral Arrangements: Legitimate Business or Unethical Entrepreneurialism," *American Journal of Law and Medicine* 15:1, pp. 61-109.

McGuire, Thomas G. and Mark V. Pauly. 1991. "Physician Response to Fee Changes With Multiple Payers," *Journal of Health Economics* 10, pp. 385-410.

McKeown, Thomas. 1988. *The Origins of Human Disease.* Oxford: Basil Blackwell.

____. 1979. *The Role of Medicine: Dream, Mirage or Nemesis?*. Princeton: Princeton University Press.

McKinlay, John B. and Sonja M. McKinlay. 1977. *Milbank Memorial Fund Quarterly* (Summer), pp. 405-428.

McMenamin, Peter. 1988. "A Crime Story From Medicare Part B," *Health Affairs* 7:5 (Winter), pp. 94-101.

Melnick, R. Shep. 1990. "The Politics of the New Property: Welfare Rights in Congress and the Courts," *Liberty, Property, and the Future of Constitutional Development.* (eds. Paul and Dickman). Albany: State University of New York Press, pp. 199-240.

Menken, Mathew. 1983. "Consequences of an Oversupply of Medical Specialists: The Case of Neurology," *New England Journal of Medicine* 308:20 (May 19), pp. 1224-1226.

Menzel, Paul T. 1990. *Strong Medicine: The Ethical Rationing of Health Care.* New York: Oxford University Press.

Mill, John Stuart. 1992. *On Liberty and Other Essays* (ed. Gray) Oxford: Oxford University Press.

Mitchell, Alanna. 1992. "Abortion Foes Hope for Victory in Saskatchewan," *Globe and Mail* (Wednesday, May 6), p. A1.

Mitchell, Janet B., William B. Stason, Kathleen A. Calore, Marc P. Frieman, and Helene T. Hewes. 1987. "Are Some Surgical Procedures Overpaid?" *Health Affairs* 6:2 (Summer), pp. 121-131.

Mitchell, Jean M. and Elton Scott. 1992. "New Evidence of the Prevalence and Scope of Physician Joint Ventures," *Journal of the American Medical Association* 268:1 (July 1), pp. 80-84.

____. 1992. "Physician Ownership of Physical Therapy Services," *Journal of the American Medical Association* 268:15 (October 21), pp. 2055-2059.

Mitchell, Jean M. and Jonathan H. Sunshine. 1992. "Consequences of Physicians' Ownership of Health Care Facilities: Joint Ventures in Radiation Therapy," *New England Journal of Medicine* 327 (November 19), pp. 1497-1501.

Mitchell, Samuel A. 1988. "Defending the U.S. Approach to Health Spending," *Health Affairs* 7:5 (Winter), pp. 31-34.

Moore *v* Regents of California. 1990. 271 California Reporter pp. 146-190.

Morgenson, Gretchen. 1991. "The Doctors and the Dealmakers," *Forbes* (April 15), pp. 38-39.

Morris, Christopher. 1991. "Moral Standing and Rational-Choice Contractarianism," *Contractarianism and Rational Choice* (ed. Vallentyne). Cambridge: Cambridge University Press, pp. 76-95.

Moyer, M. Eugene. 1989. "A Revised Look at the Number of Uninsured Americans," *Health Affairs* 8:2 (Summer), pp. 102-111.

Mueller, Dennis C. 1987. "Voting Paradox," *Democracy and Public Choice*, (Charles K. Rowley, ed.). New York: Basil Blackwell. pp. 77-102.

Nagel, Thomas. 1986. *The View From Nowhere*. New York: Oxford University Press.

Narveson, Jan. 1988. *The Libertarian Idea*. Philadelphia: Temple University Press.

Navarro, V. 1984. "A Critique of the Ideological and Political Position of the Brandt Report and the Alma-Ata Declaration," *International Journal of Health Services* 14:2 (1984), pp. 159-172.

Nelson, Robin. 1992. "Computers Tap Into Multiple Medical Information Sources," *Medical Tribune* 33:15 (August 6) p. 17.

Neuhauser, Duncan. 1990. "The Six Stool Guiac Test, A Reply," *Journal of Health Economics* 9, pp. 493-494.

_____. 1980. "Letter to the Editor: Reply to Nicholas Prescott *et al*," *New England Journal of Medicine* 303:22 (November 27), pp. 1306-1307.

Neuhauser, Duncan and Ann M. Lewicki. 1975. "What Do We Gain From the Sixth Stool Guiac?" *New England Journal of Medicine* 293:5 (July 31), pp. 226-228.

Neuschler, Edward. 1990. *Canadian Health Care: The Implications of Public Health Insurance*. Health Insurance Association of America.

Newhouse, Joseph P., Geffrey Anderson, and Leslie L. Roos.

1988. "Hospital Spending in the United States and Canada: A Comparison," *Health Affairs* 7:5 (Winter), pp. 6-16.

Nozick, Robert. 1974. *Anarchy, State, and Utopia.* New York: Basic Books.

Onwuachi-Saunders, E. Chulwudi, Deborah A. Lambert, Polly A. Marchbanks, Patrick W. O'Carroll, and James A. Mercy. 1989. "Firearm-Related Assaults on Los Angeles Roadways," *Journal of the American Medical Association* 262:16 (October 27), pp. 2262-2264.

Pauly, Mark V. 1988. "Is Medical Care Different? Old Questions, New Answers," *Journal of Health Politics, Policy and Law* 13:2 (Summer), 227-237.

Peden, Edgar A. and Mei Lin Lee. 1991. "Output and Inflation Components of Medical Care and Other Spending Changes," *Health Care Financing Review* 13:2 (Winter), pp. 75-81.

Pence, Gregory E. 1990. *Classic Cases in Medical Ethics.* New York: McGraw-Hill Publishing Company.

Perlman, Mark. 1974. "Economic History and Health Care in Industrialized Nations," *The Economics of Health and Medical Care* (ed. Perlman). New York: John Wiley & Sons, pp. 21-33.

Pfaff, Martin. 1990. "Differences in Health Care Spending Across Countries: Statistical Evidence," *Journal of Health Politics, Policy and Law* 15:1 (Spring), pp. 1-67.

Picard, Andre. 1992. "Health Budget Slashed," *Globe and Mail* (Saturday, May 9), p. A5.

Pogge, Thomas W. 1989. *Realizing Rawls.* Ithaca: Cornell University Press.

Pope, Gregory C. and John E. Schneider. 1992. "Trends in Physician Incomes," *Health Affairs* 11:1 (Spring), pp. 181-193.

Prescott, Nicholas, Kilim McPherson, and John Bell. 1980. "Letter to the Editor: Cost Effectiveness of Screening for Occult Blood in the Stool, Another Look," *New England Journal of Medicine* 303:22 (November 27), 1980.

Rakich, Jonathan S. 1991a. "Canada's Universal-Comprehensive Healthcare System," *Hospital Topics* 69:2 (Spring), pp. 14-19.

____. 1991b. "The Canadian and U.S. Health Care Systems: Profiles and Policies," *Hospital and Health Services Administration* 36:1 (Spring), pp. 25-42.

Rakich, Jonathan S. and Edmund R. Becker. 1992. "United

States Physician Payment Reform: Background and Comparison With the Canadian Model," *Health Care Management Review* 17:1, pp. 9-19.

Rankin, James W. and Bruce A. Hubbard. 1984. "Private Credentialing of Health Care: A Pragmatic Response to Academic Theory," *American Journal of Law and Medicine* 10:2 (Summer), pp. 189-200.

Rawls, John. 1988. "The Priority of Right and Ideas of the Good," *Philosophy & Public Affairs* 17, pp. 251-276.

___. 1987. "The Idea of an Overlapping Consensus," Oxford *Journal of Legal Studies* 7, pp. 1-25.

___. 1985. "Justice as Fairness: Political not Metaphysical," *Philosophy & Public Affairs* 14, pp. 223-251.

___. 1982. "The Basic Liberties and Their Priority," *Tanner Lecture on Human Values* Vol. III. Salt Lake City: University of Utah Press.

___. 1971. *A Theory of Justice*. Cambridge: Harvard University Press.

Record, Jane Cassel and Michael McCally, Stuart O. Schweitzer, Robert M. Bloomquist, and Benjamin D. Berger. 1980. "New Health Professionals After a Decade and a Half: Delegation, Productivity and Costs in Primary Care," *Journal of Politics, Policy and Law* 5:3 (Fall), pp. 470-497.

Reich, Charles A. 1965. "Individual Rights and Social Welfare: The Emerging Legal Issues" 74 *The Yale Law Journal* 1245.

___. 1964. "The New Property" 73 *The Yale Law Journal* 728.

Reinhardt, Uwe E. 1987. "Resource Allocation in Health Care: The Allocation of Lifestyles to Providers," *The Milbank Quarterly* 65:2, pp. 153-176.

___. 1985. "The Theory of Physician-Induced Demand After a Decade," *Journal of Health Economics* 4:2 (June), pp. 187-193.

Rice, Thomas H. 1987. "Induced Demand -- Can We Ever Know Its Extent?," *Journal of Health Economics* 6:4 (December), pp. 375- 376.

Rice, Thomas H. and Roberta J. Labelle. 1989. "Do Physicians Induce Demand for Medical Services?" *Journal of Health Politics, Policy and Law* 14:3 (Fall), pp. 587-600.

Robert, David. 1992. "Saskatchewan Raises Taxes to Offset Deficit," *Globe and Mail* (Friday, May 8), p. A1.

Robyn, Dorothy and Jack Hadley. 1980. "National Health Insurance and the New Health Occupations: Nurse Practitioners and Physicians' Assistants," *Journal of Health Politics, Policy and Law* 5:3 (Fall), pp. 447-469.

Ropp, Leland, Paul Visintainer, Jane Uman, and David Treloar. 1992. "Death in the City: An American Childhood Tragedy," *Journal of the American Medical Association* 267:21 (June 3), pp. 2905- 2910.

Rosenbach, Margo L. and Ashley G. Stone. 1990. "Malpractice Insurance Costs and Physician Practice," *Health Affairs* 9:4 (Winter), pp. 176-185.

Rotham, David J. 1991. *Strangers at the Bedside: A History of How Law and Bioethics Transformed Medical Decision Making.* New York: Basic Books.

Rublee, Dale A. 1989. "Medical Technology in Canada, Germany, and the United States," *Health Affairs* 8:3 (Fall), pp. 178-181.

Rutkow, Ira M. 1987. "Surgical Operations and Supply: Assessing Future Quality," *Health Affairs* 6:3 (Fall), pp. 82-89.

Sakala, Carol. 1990. "The Development of National Medical Care Programs in the United Kingdom and Canada: Applicability to Current Conditions in the United States," *Journal of Health Politics, Policy and Law* 15:4 (Winter), pp. 709-753.

Schieber, George J. 1990. "Health Expenditures in Major Industrialized Countries, 1960-87," *Health Care Financing Review* 11:4 (Summer), pp. 159-167.

Schieber, George J. and Jean-Pierre Poullier. 1988. "International Health Expenditures and Utilization Trends," *Health Affairs* 7:4 (Fall), pp. 105-117.

Schmidtz, David. 1991. *The Limits of Government: An Essay on the Public Goods Argument.* Boulder: Westview Press.

Schwartz, Leroy L. 1991. "The Medical Costs of America's Social Ills," *Wall Street Journal* (Monday, June 24), p. A10.

Sheeline, William E. 1991. "Taking on Public Enemy No. 1," *Fortune* (July 1), pp. 58-59.

Sheils, John F., Gary J. Young, and Robert Rubin. 1992. "O Canada: Do We Expect Too Much From Its Health Care System?" *Health Affairs* 11:1 (Spring), pp. 7-20.

Singer, Peter. 1981. "Altruism and Commerce: A Defense of

Titmuss Against Arrow," *Medicine and Moral Philosophy* (ed. Cohen, Nagel, and Scanlon). Princeton: Princeton University Press, pp. 159-167.

Sloan, Frank A., Joseph Valvona, James M. Perrin, and Killard W. Adamache. 1986. "Diffusion of Surgical Technology: An Exploratory Study," *Journal of Health Economics* 5:1 (March), pp. 31-61.

Slote, Michael. 1989. *Beyond Optimizing: A Study of Rational Choice*. Cambridge: Harvard University Press.

Smith, Lee. 1991. "A Cure for What Ails Medical Care," *Fortune* (July 1), pp. 44-49.

Sonnefeld, Sally T., Daniel R. Waldo, Jeffrey A. Lemieux, and David R. McKusick. 1991. "Projections of National Health Expenditures Through the Year 2000," *Health Care Financing Review* 13: 1 (Fall), pp. 1-27.

Southby, Richard F., and Jonathan S. Rakich. 1991. "International Healthcare Expenditures: Spending Totals and Public Satisfaction Among the OECD Nations," *Hospital Topics* (Spring), pp. 8-13.

Stano, Miron. 1987. "A Further Analysis of the Physician Inducement Controversy," *Journal of Health Economics* 6:3 (September), pp. 227-238.

___. 1985. "An Analysis of the Evidence on Competition in the Physician Services Markets," *Journal of Health Economics* 4:3 (September), pp. 197-211.

Starr, Paul. 1982. *The Social Transformation of American Medicine*. NY: Basic Books.

Stern, Lawrence. 1983. "Opportunity and Health Care: Criticisms and Suggestions" *Journal of Medicine and Philosophy* 8:4 (November), pp. 339-361.

Stevenson, H. Michael, A. Paul Williams, and Eugene Vayda. 1988. "Medical Politics and Canadian Medicare: Professional Response to the Canada Health Act," *The Milbank Quarterly* 66:1, pp. 65-104.

Stoeckle, John D. 1988. "Reflections on Modern Doctoring," *The Milbank Quarterly* 66:Supp. 2, pp. 76-91.

Stout, Hilary. 1992a. "Elderly Now Spend Over Twice as Much on Health as They Did Before Medicare," *Wall Street Journal* (February 26), p. B5.

___. 1992b. "Americans' Health Improves but Blacks Suffer

Higher Death Rates Than Whites," *Wall Street Journal* (Friday, June 26), p. B6.

Sugden, Robert. 1990. "Contractarianism and Norms," *Ethics* 100:4 (July) pp. 768-786.

Sumner, L. W. 1987. *The Moral Foundation of Rights.* Oxford: Oxford University Press.

Swedlow, A. *et al.* 1992. "Increased Costs and Rates of Use in the California Workers' Compensation System as a Result of Self-referral by Physicians," *New England Journal of Medicine* 327 (November 19), pp. 1522-1524.

Taylor. Malcolm G. 1987. *Health Insurance and Canadian Public Policy: The Seven Decisions That Created the Canadian Health Insurance System and Their Outcomes* 2nd ed. Toronto: Institute of Public Administration of Canada.

____. 1986. "The Canadian Health Care System 1974-1984," *Medicare At Maturity.* (eds. Evans and Stoddart). Calgary: The University of Calgary Press, pp. 3-39.

____. 1978. *Health Insurance and Canadian Public Policy: The Seven Decisions That Created the Canadian Health Insurance System.* Montreal: McGill-Queen's University Press.

Temin, Peter. 1983. "Costs and Benefits in Switching Drugs From Rx to OTC," *Journal of Health Economics* 2:3 (December), pp. 187-205.

"Texas Near End of Psychiatric Hospital Chain Probe." 1992. *American Medical News* (July 6/13), p. 56.

Titmuss, Richard. 1971. *The Gift Relationship.* NY: Vintage Books.

Todd, James S. 1992. "Must the Law Assure Ethical Behavior?" *Journal of the American Medical Association* 268:1 (July 1), p. 98.

Vallentyne, Peter. 1991. "Contractarianism and the Assumption of Mutual Unconcern," *Contractarianism and Rational Choice* (ed. Vallentyne). New York: Cambridge University Press, pp. 71-75.

Van Alstyne, William. 1977. "Cracks in 'The New Property': Adjudicating Due Process in the Administrative State," 62 *Cornell Law Review* 445.

Van Loon, Richard. 1986. "Canadian Perspective: Learning From Our Experience," *Medicare at Maturity: Achievements, Lessons and Challenges* (eds. Evans and Stoddart). Calgary: The University of Calgary Press, pp. 451-472.

Waldholz, Michael. 1991. "Computer 'Brain' Outperforms Doctors in Diagnosing Heart Attacks," *Wall Street Journal* (Monday, December 2), p. A7.

Walker, Michael. 1992. "Cold Reality: How They Don't Do It in Canada," *Reason* (March), pp. 35-39.

___. 1989. "Canada is no Health Care Model," *Human Events* (December 23), p. 9.

___. 1988. "Neighborly Advice on Health Care," *Wall Street Journal* (June 8), p. 24.

Wedig, Gerald, Janet B. Mitchell, and Jerry Cromwell. 1989. "Can Price Controls Induce Optimal Physician Behavior?" *Journal of Health Politics, Policy and Law* 14:3 (Fall), pp. 601-620.

Weil, Thomas P. 1991. The U.S. Healthcare System After NHI," *Hospital Topics* 69:2 (Spring), pp. 36-40.

Weiler, Paul C., Joseph P. Newhouse, and Howart H. Hiatt. 1992. "Proposal for Medical Liability Reform," *Journal of the American Medical Association* 267:17 (May 6), pp. 2355-2358.

Weisbrod, Burton A. 1991. "The Health Care Quadrilemma: An Essay on Technological Change, Insurance, Quality of Care, and Cost Containment," *Journal of Economic Literature* 29:2 (June), pp. 523- 552.

Wellman, Carl. 1982. *Welfare Rights*. Totowa, NJ: Rowman & Allanheld.

Wicker, Tom. 1991. "A Costly 10 Percent," *New York Times* (Sunday, July 21) Section 4, p. 17.

Wikler, Daniel. 1983. "Philosophical Perspectives on Access to Health Care: An Introduction," *Securing Access to Health Care. Washington: President's Commission for the Study of Ethical Problems in Medicine and Biomedical and Behavioral Research*, pp. 119-120.

Williams, Bernard. 1985. *Ethics and the Limits of Philosophy*. Cambridge: Harvard University Press.

Winslow, Ron. 1992. "Some Overhead Costs Help Save Money," *Wall Street Journal* (Friday, June 19), p. B1.

___. 1991. "Rising Supply of Doctors May be Bad Medicine for Health Costs," *Wall Street Journal* (May 8), p. B1.

Wolinsky, Fredric D. 1988. "The Professional Dominance Perspective, Revisited," *The Milbank Quarterly* 66:Supp. 2, pp. 33-47.

Woolhandler, Steffie. and David U. Himmelstein. 1989. "A National Health Program: Northern Light at the End of the

Tunnel," *Journal of the American Medical Association* 762:15 (October 20), pp. 2136-2137.

Yett, Donald E., William Derr, Richard L. Ernst, and Joel W. Hay. 1983. "Physician Pricing and Health Insurance Reimbursement," *Health Care Financing Review* 5:2 (Winter), pp. 69-80.

York, Geoffrey. 1992a. "Medical-Services Review to Focus on Real Benefits," *Globe and Mail* (Friday, June 19), p. A4.

_____. 1992b. "Lankin Warns of Curbs on MDs," *Globe and Mail* (Tuesday, June 23), p. A5.

Index

rights: positive and negative, 3-4, 131n57
Schmidtz, D., 57, 59-60, 70, 77, 83
self-referral, 5, 9-11, 17, 103, 107, 123n9
Starr, P., 96, 99
Sumner, W., 3
straightforward maximizers, 82-83
transparent, 82-83
translucent, 82-83
veil of ignorance, 32
Wikler, D., 37